I0776334

TOXIC WORKPLACES

FROM HURT TO HEALING

ANNA REMIJN DERHAM

BALBOA.PRESS

A DIVISION OF HAY HOUSE

Balboa Press books may be ordered through booksellers or by contacting:

Balboa Press
A Division of Hay House
1663 Liberty Drive
Bloomington, IN 47403
www.balboapress.com.au
AU TFN: 1 800 844 925 (Toll Free inside Australia)
AU Local: 0283 107 086 (+61 2 8310 7086 from outside Australia)

ISBN: 978-1-9822-9042-9 (sc)
ISBN: 978-1-9822-9043-6 (e)

Print information available on the last page.

Balboa Press rev. date: 05/13/2021

Contents

Chapter 1   Giselle – Working for the dragon narcissist 1

Chapter 2   Dulce working for the Corporate Psychopath 10

Chapter 3   Debbie – The force of destruction..22

Chapter 4   Turquoise – Men at work misbehaving..25

Chapter 5   Destiny – You get what you focus on, so focus on what you want 36

Chapter 6   Turquoise – Men at work misbehaving; from hurt to healing..............................59

Chapter 7   Debbie – The force of destruction; from hurt to healing 73

Chapter 8   Dulce – working for the Corporate Psychopath; from hurt to healing.................78

Chapter 9   Giselle – Working for the dragon narcissist; from hurt to healing 91

Acknowledgements...103

Giselle – Working for the dragon narcissist

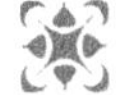

Beware of the Crocodile, who pretends to be a paragon of goodness and purity. This saintly exterior is a front for the Crocodile's drive for power, attention and sensual appetite.

– Unknown.

"And as the bad guys dispose of their dead bodies in the mangroves for the Crocodile to ravish and spew out their indigestion, the Crabs patiently wait to devour the leftover so keep out of the mangroves," warns Giselle's inner voice.

Giselle's hands are sweating, and her heart is pumping faster than usual. She clicks the red button on her phone. She draws in a deep breath and exhales noisily.

"I would rather be home with my dog," mumbles Giselle.

Thinking of her dog cheers her somewhat as she imagines stroking her dog, Jack's soft coat and giving Jack the cuddles that he so loves. The more Giselle reflects on the good feelings she gets from sharing the love and drawing in Jack's unconditional loving energy, the more it makes her smile.

"That's right, Jack's no judgement, and judgement-free power is the energy that I need right now, and yet I have to return to the mangroves for a meeting with the dragon narcissist whose name is Delilah. I reckon Delilah blows venomous gas through her nostrils, and her breath smells like acetone," mumbles Giselle as she wipes the tears from her eyes and hangs on to the stair railings to steady herself.

"What was I thinking to attract yet another intimidation experience in the workplace?" Giselle quietly asks herself,

"I love the excitement of adventure in my life, but choosing another workplace with narcissistic behaviour is a bit too much of an adventure for me right now. As much as I try, I just can't connect with Delilah, and then the other staff become afraid of connecting with me because they fear her wrath.

"Every day, Delilah tells me that I am not to befriend any of the staff whilst I am at work or out of work hours," Giselle mutters.

"An even more significant value to me is connection because I like connecting with people even more than adventure, but what do I have to do for people in these places to like me so I can connect with them? It doesn't matter what I do. I'm always wrong. It seems to me that the more she tells me I'm wrong, the more the others in my workplace perceive me as incompetent," mumbles Giselle as she walks towards her car.

Feelings of being wrong are energetically building within her, and Giselle realises it is time to speak with a professional Counsellor.

"It doesn't matter what I do. Delilah always tells me it's wrong. I try hard to please Delilah, and I do what I believe she wants of me," Giselle rubs her forehead and squints and then continues ranting to her Counsellor,

"Delilah delegates jobs to me where she watches and waits, and then when the time is right, she attacks and tells me that I'm doing it wrong and it has to be correct, according to her. Delilah just gives me the job with a partial description of the expected outcome, and then I hear her on the phone giving tasks to her Crabs that she carefully talks them through. She makes every effort to explain each and every detail carefully. When I ask for more information, she tells me that I should just know. I can draw on my successes in my previous experience, but that is someone else's right, not Delilah's right.

That's when I remember the stories that I have heard about the mangroves where I have a vision of crocodiles and Crabs sitting in the mangroves waiting expectantly. I imagine the story where the crocodiles and Crabs clear the mangroves of any evidence for the bad guys and the Delilahs in this world who get away with dumping their baggage. I can hear my imagined bad guys threatening and intimidating those around them and then tossing those around them into the mangroves to disable them from telling anyone of the pain and gaps created in their lives," Giselle stops talking to sip her water and then continues,

"In my opinion, Delilah is one of those people who swiftly scale the corporate ladder. It seems that she projects her feelings of inadequacy onto the level of staff one rung below her, which includes me. I know that my colleagues and I feel disempowered, and our productivity is falling because we're confused, and we all fear her venom. She is driving us towards her creation of a dysfunctional workspace.

On the other hand, Delilah charms her supervisors, who congratulate her for a job well done. How does that work?" Giselle asks her Counsellor, who is still in the listening mode because Giselle's Counsellor can't get a word in edgeways. Giselle continues,

"You know right now, Delilah seems to have lost sight of the big picture and the outcomes that she once aspired to. It's like she's confused because she's lost her way. She doesn't seem to know where she's going and how she will get there."

Giselle's Counsellor continues to take notes and then observes Giselle in her Silence. After the Silence, Giselle sits upright. She lifts her eyes to focus on the light fitting on the wall that sits just above her direct line of sight. Sitting quietly with her eyes raised, Giselles creates space to sort through her thoughts. When she is ready, Giselle begins speaking again,

"I think that Delilah, my dragon narcissist's feet are stuck in the mud, and each movement seems to suck her down even more. She spends her time concentrating on specific details and delegates the rest. I try hard to do the right thing, and I search for solutions based on what has worked in my past workplaces, but every time firing from her nostrils, she shoots me down and each time I burn and scar."

Giselle falls silent again as she sorts through her thoughts before continuing her speak,

"Delilah was nice to me in the beginning, and then wham, Delilah turned on me. Her micromanagement methods intensified, and she always holds me responsible for everything that she believes is wrong in her department. I can't do anything right."

Giselle lifts her eyes and focuses on her chosen spot on the wall again, which seems to give her time to refocus. When Giselle is ready, she continues,

"I remember that time I rang to let her know that I wasn't well enough to come into work, only to be told not to return to work until I was resilient." Giselle falls silent again and feels anger rise within her. Her stomach churns, and her breathing shortens. She isn't sure that she can speak, and then she does,

"Resilient for what? Other staff can return from sick leave on a rehabilitation plan as needed. I have to ask the question. Why was I commanded to be resilient and then excluded from having a rehabilitation plan designed for my return?"

Giselle sits quietly whilst she composes herself to continue speaking,

"Delilah likes to knock me down and watch me flounder, and as I begin to get up, she knocks me down even more fiercely. It seems to me that Delilah really is a dragon narcissist Crocodile, focusing on its prey. She targets me to unnerve me, just like the mangrove Crocodile that waits with jaws wide open ready to snap. Delilah is that dragon narcissist Crocodile with her army of Crabs waiting by her side, waiting for her to feed them the leftovers."

Giselle shivers and then draws in a deep breath to ground herself and then continues,

"I feel claustrophobic and closed in like a prisoner held against my will. I need to get out of the mangroves where my dragon narcissist Crocodile holds me captive. I feel like she is hiding in the density of the mangroves, observing me and waiting for her opportunity to snap her jaws shut to chomp me up and spit me out. She is destroying my whole life as I know it."

Giselle takes another deep breath and exhales as she pushes back her long blond hair from her face. Her piercing blue eyes fill with angry tears. She steadies herself by peering at the light fitting on the wall and then says,

"Think I need to escape these mangroves where I work with my dragon narcissist before the mangroves become my burial ground. She stroked my ego when first we met, then she stood back and observed me to learn what triggers my insecurities as she prepares me for the snapping of her jaws to chomp me up, spit me out and leave my leftovers for her Crabs to feast on."

Giselle stops and rubs her eyes and then continues talking,

"I have always got my jobs on merit. No one hands them to me on a plate. I apply, I participate in the interview and any other required processes to prove my worth to confirm my suitability for the position, and I got this one the same way, but I need to leave this job. When I think about it, I realise that this is the first job where I lost my mojo to either study areas of interest or work a second job out of work hours. Never before have I jumped straight into bed after work. I mean that I walk through the front door, close it behind me, drop my work clothes on the floor, put my pyjama's on and jump into bed for the night, and I have done this many times in the last few weeks. I feel like my energy is draining more and more every day."

Giselle stops to catch her breath, and then Giselle wipes the tears from her eyes then says,

"I have been working on my resume, speaking with people linked to the same industry in other institutions and watching the job ads."

"I think that you have already decided, and in your mind, you have already left," says Giselle's Counsellor.

"I haven't left yet," says Giselle,

"But I know that I will leave, and I know that I need to leave on my terms, and I know that I need help to build my confidence to do that."

Giselle stops to take some deep breaths. Then Giselle raises her eyes and stares at her chosen spot on the wall to contemplate. She feels like she has been staring for hours and long enough to feel a sense of calm wrap around her, and then Giselle remembers a time when she did feel confident. Her mind fills with memories and thoughts. She wrinkles her brow and narrows her eyes as she reflects on everything she has gotten through and how she had the strength to push through even the most challenging happenings. Images of the horrific, fatal car crash swept through her mind and then she remembered how her life had stopped and changed in one split second. That one split second that buried her dreams and left her all alone to navigate another life. Giselle had mourned her loss, she had cried, she had withdrawn, she had learned her strength, and like the phoenix, she rose from the ashes and made another life for herself because she knew there was no going back. Giselle had moved through these phases with confidence and wonders why can't she do that now?

"I feel stuck. Delilah is a block that I can't get over, can't get under and can't get around,"

Giselle bemoans and stops to breathe deeply whilst digging deep to find her intestinal fortitude or courage to speak her truth. Giselle feels a redness creeping up her neck and her gut constricting, and then she says,

"I feel like Delilah squashes me with her constant criticism of me. I feel like I am drowning in my perceived loss of competence as a functional human being. I need help to find my strength to be like the phoenix and rise from the ashes. I need help to re-discover my belief in myself to know that I can survive the time I need until I can successfully secure another more suitable job for me."

Giselle's Counsellor acknowledges Giselle for her courage and searches for a way to help Giselle.

"Maybe it is about fitting in instead of trying to belong," Giselle's Counsellor says quietly whilst observing Giselle's reaction, then continues,

"Some people are thinkers, and some people feel their way through their lives. Giselle, would you agree that you feel your way through life and perhaps take on others energy?"

"Yes, I think I do absorb other people's energies,"

Giselle pauses for a moment and then continues,

"When Delilah tells me sad stories about her family or tells me about people she knows that affect her adversely, I feel sorry for her," responds Giselle.

"Would it be fair to say that Delilah is a thinker and sometimes overthinks before she speaks?" asks Giselle's Counsellor.

"Maybe. Sometimes, I notice that Delilah leads with her head forward, leaving her heart lagging behind her head, and I believe that means that she disconnects her head from her heart space. I have heard others say that they believe that Delilah lacks emotional intelligence.

I've heard that stress and anxiety reduce concentration and that long term stress can cause a decline in cognitive functions. I understand that stress triggers cortisol and adrenalin, stimulating the sympathetic nervous system draining blood away from the brain towards the body's fighting parts, which is the fight or flight response. I can wish that Delilah will fly away like a graceful swan. However, I know that Delilah will stay and fight because sometimes it seems that she becomes anxious and stressed when she assimilates as a high performing woman who takes her estrogen and changes it to testosterone. Kind of like she androgynises herself to become an alpha something, a narcissistic alpha something, to hide her incompetence. It seems that even though Delilah has the learned knowledge, she has reached a level where she is out of her depth with trying to apply her knowledge."

Giselle looks around and raises her hand to cover her mouth. Taking a breath, she removes her hand to exhale and asks,

"Where did that come from?"

Giselle sits upright in her chair and then continues,

"I have noticed that Delilah stops momentarily to think before she speaks, sometimes momentarily and sometimes for longer moments."

Giselle stops talking and looks down at her feet. Giselle's Counsellor gives Giselle time to think and then says,

"Keep in mind that thinkers use more energy to feel, and people who feel their way through life take more energy to think and both sustain their natural energies more easily. When events escalate, and people feel out of control of their event, they can become overwhelmed and see what's in front of them using only their natural energies. Can you step into Delilah's shoes and pretend to be a thinker to see things from her perspective?" asks Giselle's Counsellor.

Giselle takes a deep breath, smiles and nods. Giselle's Counsellor continues,

"I can share with you a memory. A time that I remember when my Mentor emphasised the importance of understanding differences in people's values, beliefs, priorities, motivations and expectations, and that is what makes the differences because they shape everyone differently."

Giselle squints her clear blue eyes and tilts her head to listen even more. Giselle's Counsellor continues,

"And there are root causes or events that will have occurred in a person's past that has caused the creation of today's irrational conflicts. My Mentor told me of specific reactions where people became stuck behind their belief in their rightness. They were right, and everyone who disagreed was wrong. Other people sabotage their actions because they aim for perfection, and perfection in a world of imperfections doesn't exist. I can share with you that perfectionists who set impossibly high standards for others can tend to be narcissistic and lack the emotional intelligence you spoke about earlier. It appears that they don't care about fitting in or belonging. I wonder that if you may be able to step into Delilah's shoes to give you a greater understanding of why she does what she does. Do you think that would be helpful, and more so, do you think you could manage that?"

Giselle thinks for a moment and then responds,

"You know, I think I can try to do that. Maybe if I see things from Delilah's perspective, I will understand what she wants from me and know what to deliver or know when not to respond. Yes, I think that I can do that for the time that I have left here whilst I find my forever job."

Giselle leaves the building feeling lighter with a skip in her step and hope for the way forward.

"Yes, I can do this because I have pleased others and obeyed rules and regulations in my past. I can do it again," Giselle Mumbles quietly to herself.

Her mobile phone rings, interrupting her musings on her walk from the Counsellor's office to her car. Giselle jumps because she is immersed in her thinking and celebrating her aha moments from her counselling session. Excited expectation quickly becomes a heavy burden as she hears the dragon narcissist's voice,

"Do not return to work unless you bring your resilience with you. Make sure you return to work with your resilience intact, and we are meeting in fifteen minutes," are the last commanding words that Giselle hears through her brand new mobile phone. How quickly Giselle's feelings of lightness and happiness dissolve.

"How did my dragon narcissist know that I was leaving my Counsellor's office just ten minutes down the road from the office?" Giselle asks herself.

Giselle has fifteen minutes to get back in time for her meeting. She can feel the weight of a heavy burden build even more within her. Giselle can't lift her feet because her shoes feel like they are as heavy as lead. She can feel her heart thump loudly in her chest and feel the sweat pouring from her. Giselle wipes her hand down the leg of her work pants to take away the sticky, damp feeling. She wants to run, but she knows that she has to get back in time for her meeting.

"I feel like my outside environment is growing heavy to meet the heaviness feeling within me," retorts Giselle.

Giselle notices that the sky above is as dark as night with a vivid green tinge in the grey clouds. The thunderclaps are loud and becoming even more piercing, like a waterfall of electricity falling from the skies. Giselle wipes away the tears that fall on her cheeks, then yelps,

"I feel even more overwhelmed with lightning spears whistling past me and the thunderclaps booming above me. I can't move my feet. I feel the fear inside me as I reflect on seeing myself as the dragon narcissist Crocodile's prey. I can see the Crocodile watching me with mouth wide open ready to snap shut to chomp me up and spit me out. I remember her words that resonate in my head. Do not return to work until you are resilient."

Giselle's internal voices are talking over her cacophony of thoughts, telling her,

"Do not to do anything because I can't do, I can't do anything, so stay safe and don't do anything."

Giselle had heard that advice before,

"And most of all, don't let them see you cry."

Giselle's ego is working hard to keep her safe by keeping her the same. Her feet are stuck, her body is rigid, and she can't move.

"I remember that I learned how to change my focus that changed my thoughts to feel anticipated excitement when I was a young girl sitting in church. The words that I heard from the pulpit were angry in tone and seemed like threats of hellfire and damnation, and those words scared me. I was required to attend church every Sunday and often twice on a Sunday, and I did so to please my mother. I would sit in church next to my mother and tune out. I would plan adventures where I imagined myself laughing, moving, and enjoying my imaginary friends and imagined surroundings. Sometimes I would smell the aroma of burnt sugar as we made toffees, or I imagined that I could taste the delectable homemade ice cream portions where I could feel saliva build in my mouth. That is when I would wriggle in my seat to stop me drooling, and then I would catch the tone of the sermons, which spewed out threats of hellfire and damnation scared me so much that I wanted to run. The spokesperson was an Irish man who lamented the trouble in Northern Ireland where his friends and family lived. It was a time of political and sectarian violence in Northern Ireland that fuelled the long sermons that the religious speaker presented from his pulpit. The religious speaker's distressful tonality and fearful words were often enough to automatically trigger me to retreat into the safety of my imagination. My mother would tell me that all good strong little girls were required to sit still and listen, and that's what I looked like I was doing," murmurs Giselle's internal voice,

"I'm a grown woman now and find it more difficult to distract myself from the words that I receive as I find I internalise others words even more because now I am in the habit of wanting to please people even more, so I make an effort to listen. And as I filter in those words as mine, then I feel like crying, and if I cry, I know that Delilah will go in even more to terrorise me, and then I will feel even more hopeless and more helpless."

Thoughts career through Giselle's mind, and then she speaks out loud,

"So many thoughts, which one do I concentrate on?"

Giselle senses her focus change because Delilah's demands for resilience effectively generate a shift within her. She focuses on her thinking around resilience, and she senses that power within her that lets her change her thoughts as she did as a child sitting in church. Giselle remembered feeling frightened. Then she remembered feeling her fear dissipate, leaving her space to change her thoughts from being frightened to imagining the experience of excited anticipation of experiencing the fun she imagined. Giselle remembered thinking about the fun she had riding her bike and the freedom that it gave her. Giselle remembered visualising her experience of learning how to ride. Giselle sensed her resilience when she fell and got up, and when she fell again, she got up again because her motivation was strong to know that she would experience the freedom and adventure that her bike rides gave her.

"How do I do resilience now and still please Delilah?" asks Giselle, and then says,

"I have survived worse experiences than Delilah. I feel like part of me knows that I feel like I am on a painful downward spiral when I separate from my emotions. If I push my feelings down, they rise within me at the least expected moments, and then I feel out of control. As a young person, I remember I experienced immersing in my emotions without building a story. I discovered that when I can let my emotions pass, then I have a sense of control over my feelings and emotions. When I permitted my fearful emotions to release, I felt relieved. I remember that feeling after my car accident that stole my dreams. I couldn't influence the car crash because it had happened. I remember that I discovered that I could affect how I felt when I controlled what I thought. I remember sensing then that my feelings that I create from my thoughts were the most critical thing in my life because that is all I had left," says Giselle,

"I want to do that again. I just need to find my confidence and courage to do that. I want to have the confidence to believe in me, to feel free to choose my emotional well-being to choose how I respond when I feel my emotions. I want to find my confidence to feel my fearful emotions, acknowledge them and then watch them leave me like visitors do when their visit finishes,"

Giselle stops to take a breath, a sip of her water and then continues,

"Another part of me wants to please others, and then I listen to them whilst taking on their emotions. When Delilah's wrath hits me, it hits hard. I feel her anger and feel my fear expand. Sometimes I feel emotions and wonder from where they came. I try to please the dragon narcissist, but she always tells me that I am not good enough to work with her. She seems to undermine everything that I do until I start believing that I am not good enough. I feel like a young child who has stolen ice cream from the freezer even though she knows that she will be severely disciplined if she is found out. And as I question my fear of not being good enough and my fear of being found out, I can feel my self-doubt build even more. I feel stuck, helpless and hopeless. That's when I can no longer find the courage or the strength within me to fight back, and each time I feel even more useless."

Giselle stops to listen to her Counsellor's who says,

"Now that we have discovered what your challenges are, I suggest that you seek a Hypnotherapist to coach and guide you in self-hypnosis to make your desired changes even more quickly. When you change your focus to believe in yourself, you will find the strength to be a better version of you to create a vision of a better work environment and work towards attracting that environment. You may even discover how to change your strategies to cope with your current workplace. A Coach and Hypnotherapist can lead you to choose your choice for your change around the way you think about habits that hold you back. Hypnotherapy can help you overcome obstacles to lead you towards becoming the best version of you to empower you to overcome obstacles along the way. A Hypnotherapist can guide you to identify your blocks and guide you through them. A Hypnotherapist can mentor you and guide you to visualise a workplace of choice where you feel confident to apply because you sense it to be a comfortable fit. A Coach and Hypnotherapist can help you integrate any conflicting parts of indecision within you to resolve that conflict to give you clarity of thought in your decision making and so much more.

You can discover how to choose your choice for changing your focus that will change the meaning of events in your life and build your confidence to see things differently, and you may be able to do the same in your current environment whilst you find another environment where you fit and belong."

Giselle listens and spends time contemplating, and then she says,

"Now, I remember that I have used self-hypnosis in the past to overcome the fear of public speaking. I learned to change my focus from fearful nervousness to excited anticipation. I backed myself to find the confidence and courage to present without fearful interference. I remember how thrilled I felt afterwards when I received congratulatory feedback for my presentation. I did it once, and I can do it again. I need to recover and acknowledge that I need help, and I believe that through being guided to use self-hypnosis, I can learn to believe in myself to build my confidence to change my focus and overcome my fear of Delilah and see clearly to plan for the future,"

Giselle smiles to herself and believes that she can learn to resolve her people-pleasing habits by experiencing hypnotherapy and coaching. She can learn to enable her courage and learn to build her confidence to make space for her courage to return to support the next part of her journey.

"And here I am sitting in a comfortable chair. Let my hypnotherapy induction begin," says Giselle to Alicia, her Mentor and Hypnotherapist.

"I know that you are wondering, and it's a good thing to wonder because that means that you are learning many things, and all the things, all the things that you can learn, provide you with new insights and new understandings. And you can you know, can't you not choose your choice for your change and know it's more or less the right thing to choose? You are sitting here listening to me tell you about changing your focus to choose your thoughts to change your feelings to know that you can. And that means that your unconscious mind is also here and can hear what I say. And since that is the case, you are probably learning, and it's more or less the right thing, that you can choose from the many opportunities available to you to be the architect of your life. You already know more at an unconscious level than you think you do, and it's not right for me to tell you learn this or learn that. That's right, you learn in any way you want and in any order. You are sitting here, listening to me, and immersing in my stories."

C H A P T E R   T W O

Dulce working for the Corporate Psychopath

Different mangroves, another Crocodile, other times. The Crocodile is biting, the Crabs are following, and the mangroves are beckoning

There is not a track up the mountain because there is no mountain in this seaside country town. Dulce believes that she is on an even track with a promise of clear direction in the established and successful institution where she will be working. She remembers thinking, how lucky am I to be an employee in a thriving institution that sustainably keeps up with rapid change happening in the 21st Century. A balanced work environment with staff consistency established policies and procedures and enthusiastic staff having fun. She believes that she is well suited to support middle management with a prospect of longevity in her new position.

Business plans are in place with all the planning documents that fall from explicit instruction on how things work. There are processes and procedures to guide action taking and decision making associated with rules and regulations.

Dulce imagines that there will be variety in her new job because the institution has to move forward to remain viable. It seems that staying abreast of change and celebrating success are embedded in the new institutions' values.

"How can I go wrong?" Dulce says out loud,

"I feel like I can do this. I know I can." Dulce breathes deeply to settle the feeling of butterflies flying around in her stomach. Her nervous excitement is almost uncontainable. Dulce's sweaty palms make the steering wheel slip between her fingers.

"Concentrate. I have to park this car and get to my induction across the road. I don't want to be late on the first day of work. I'm so looking forward to my new job. Hope I fit in and can do this," Dulce says out loud inside the cabin of her car.

Dulce senses doubt creeping into her mind, and her nervous excitement becomes stippled with a little bit of anxiety when she thinks about her future. She pushes her greying hair back off her face and secures her hair with her sunglasses. Standing tall, she is ready to look the world in the eye and face her new beginning with confidence and enthusiasm.

"I know so many good people who have worked here, and some are still working here. It will be the best job of my career." Dulce assures herself as she walks across the road towards the building where she has organised to meet her new boss, Cyan.

Dulce holds her head high and a little in front of her body. As if she is moving forward with a strong-willed intellect whilst disconnecting her brain from her heart space where her emotional intelligence lives. Dulce can feel a growing pain in her neck stretch towards her head. She pulls her head back in line with her back, and the pain recedes. Dulce takes a deep breath and then grins broadly.

She opens the door and crosses the threshold, where she sees a row of seats tucked under a servery window with a sign-in book on the servery counter. Dulce signs herself in for her three-hour induction, and afterwards, she returns to the chairs and sits under the servery window.

"You must be Dulce," says the young blonde girl who is leaning out of the servery window,

"Cyan has asked that you take a seat and wait for her here. Cyan will be here shortly to welcome you and take you on a tour of your new digs."

"Thank you," says Dulce.

Thoughts race through Dulce's mind, and she remembers that she has met Cyan at a work function earlier in the year. Dulce sits quietly in her chair and imagines that she is back at that work function. Familiar faces surround her, and then Dulce sees Cyan. She is the unsociable human form sitting on a solitary chair at the back of the room. No matter how hard Dulce imagines, she cannot see Cyan's face because Cyan is sitting with her head bowed as she appears to focus on her feet.

"I hope I recognise her when she comes to collect me," mumbles Dulce.

Dulce feels her throat constrict and feels an impulse to cough. She looks around and is relieved to see that now she is the only person in the room. She drinks from her water bottle and swallows the desire to cough when she hears,

"Hello. Where have you parked, Dulce?"

Dulce crosses her fingers and says,

"Hello, Cyan. I have parked in the street."

Cyan smiles and says,

"I will show you where the staff carpark is so that you can park there tomorrow. I was pleased to complete your written onsite induction and get it to you in time for your start today. It will probably take you about two years for you to settle into your new position."

Dulce is speechless. That's a first, thinks Dulce.

"Two years. How different can it be? Yes, it's a different institution, but it is within the same industry where I have always worked. Well, for the past twenty years anyway. I guess other places have different cultures and varied ways of doing things, and it would be different," Dulce mutters quietly to herself.

Cyan and Dulce pad across the road towards another building that is bordered by mangroves. Dulce knows that beyond the mangroves runs a river that flows into the sea. What she doesn't realise is this river is a place where Crocodiles breed and live.

As they walk, Dulce catches glimpses of the azure blue sea at the bottom of the road. The water sparkles and the sparkles are dancing happily all over. Dulce wants to be part of that happiness. And as Dulce shifts her focus to look back towards Cyan, Dulce feels her sparkle dull, so Dulce concentrates on the weight of carrying her induction booklets, purse, lunch, and jacket. Then Dulce decides to reassure herself and change her thinking. She mutters quietly to herself,

"I'll have time to settle in. That will help me learn the different ways of doing things, and I will have time to adjust to fit into a new culture."

Dulce settles into the silent walk with Cyan that becomes a walk with ease after experiencing information overload at her induction. She begins to feel a sense of certainty that feels comfortable and changes her focus to imagine and feel her nervous excitement reignite.

"This will be the most exciting job of my career. I believe that I will be able to develop my creativity and enhance my leadership of self and others," Dulce Mumbles quietly to herself.

Dulce knows that she has grown to become the leader she would like to lead her. She prides herself on being empathetic, service-driven and interested in what people have to say. Dulce spends more time listening than talking because her strong desire to connect with others' feelings is vital. Dulce likes to think that she can be tactful because she chooses her words carefully to avoid miscommunication. Dulce appreciates a calm environment with her team on board to meet challenges or plan for future change. She decides to believe that this institution has the right feel for her. Then her inner voice draws her attention to,

"What if they focus on my weakness, where I try to please others because I tie my self-worth to others opinion of me?" Dulce gulps because she has listened to her inner voice, ask the what-if question. Then she takes a deep breath and reassures herself when she tells herself,

"I know I will strive to meet everyone's expectations, and I know I will be motivated to do so because not meeting expectations will mean judgement and people not liking me. How can I work as part of a team of people who don't like me? I know not everyone will like me. If most of them like me, I will have a connection to build on to have a workable team environment, and besides, I want people to like me."

In time gone by, people judged Dulce for being too trusting. Sometimes she would trust first and then realise that they didn't deserve her trust, which ultimately caused her pain and sometimes got her into trouble when she trusted the wrong person. She would often overlook people's personality, strengths, quirks and weaknesses. She would watch for other people's approval, and she assumed that other people's values would match her values. Dulce remembers that a friend of a friend studying psychology said that the next occurrence will be even more challenging and likened to being hit with a heavier hammer if you don't learn from one experience. It seems that

Dulce may yet have to learn her lesson and know people first before showing her vulnerability. Then she can become more discerning to align with like-minded people to have a sense of whom she can trust.

Dulce is about to experience a hit with a heavier hammer because of her people-pleasing habit. Dulce automatically trusted Cyan to lead her and has not yet heard the rumour that Cyan has deep darkness that is well hidden in her mangrove of life. Dulce is soon to feel the hit with the heavier hammer, and she will discover her first learning in this environment. Enter at your own risk, or please do not enter the mangroves at all because Cyan, the Crocodile, will snap you, chomp you up, spit you out and only then can her Crabs devour the leftovers. The Crocodile doesn't care who you are or what you do. Cyan only cares about herself to ensure that everyone sees her shine and others dull in comparison. And these are her unwritten rules.

Rule no one.

Keep out of the mangroves unless you see the blackness and denser shadow that embodies Cyan's conscious life.

"You can't write," snaps Cyan.

Cyan's blackness and denser shadow admonishingly says,

"Do you even know what you are supposed to write?"

It doesn't take long for Dulce to think that Cyan deliberately turns the tables. Dulce's internal voice ponders her predicament,

"One minute Cyan pretends to be my best friend, and then the next minute she turns on me. Cyan treats me as an equal and turns when I least expect it. She turns to push her perception of being intellectually superior. Like the Crocodile, Cyan has a powerful bite coupled with a full-bodied twisting motion to disable and ascertain dominance and break her prey into small pieces for easy ingestion. Cyan doesn't notice the pain that she incurs, nor does she care.

Rule number two.

You do not request clarity. You have to know how to write and what words to write.

Dulce observes the change in Cyan as her eyes become slits in her face and her drooping narrow lips open, showing her yellow teeth ready to bite as she spits out the words,

"You should know what to do, what to write, and understand what my expectations are. You come here with experience, so you should just know what to do. Do not ask me again."

"I try so hard to do it right. I believe that I listen for understanding to know what words Cyan the Crocodile wants me to write. And every time, Cyan spits out her words differently each time And every time, I can feel the tears well behind my eyes. And every time, I fight to stave off my tears," says Dulce,

"Maybe she is right, and perhaps I can't do anything right in this environment. Cyan has sacrificed her family life for study and worked hard to work her way into her position," mutters Dulce.

Rule number three.

Do not care for other Wallabies and do not befriend other Wallabies.

Thoughts rush through Dulce's mind as she reflects on her values of connection, loyalty and integrity.

"Cyan doesn't care for her staff, including me, whom she calls Wallabies. She sees them as a threat, and when she becomes overwhelmed, Cyan buries herself in the detail of small incidental things and then calls Wallabies out for not meeting her demands to read her mind to meet the little arbitrary things. They, too, get into trouble for not using her exact words in their writing. Cyan will not approve projects to further the institution's way forward and blame the Wallabies for no results. Cyan always cunningly sets up others to take responsibility for her failures. She is the only one who knows how to write, and her Wallabies will not undermine her. I think Cyan likes to create confusion, sit back and watch as people reach in vain for the lifeline that she could throw to mentor them in their jobs," mumbles Dulce,

"If Cyan chooses, she will throw the lifeline and give step by step instruction to empower her Crabs on the bottom level of her structure and then demonstrate her expectations whilst telling the Wallabies who sit in between Cyan and her Crabs to do what they have to because they should know-how," Dulce reflects on her musings and then remembers when a discontented red-necked Wallaby said,

"Cyan, the Crocodile, has no emotional intelligence. That's her problem." Cyan scratches her forehead and then says,

"I'm not allowed to mix with the other Wallabies because Cyan says so, and I try so hard to please her to settle the turbulent waters. Time has passed by, and I agree that Cyan lacks emotional intelligence because she should know that my relationship with my staff would establish rapport to share ideas. If a wallaby happens to jump from the team play circle boundary into the circle boundary of friendship, then so be it, and we will still not be a threat to her. We would potentially become an even more dynamic team because of our solidarity. It's not like I'm looking for a marriage commitment because I'm already married, and my soulmate and I live exclusively within in our unconditional love circle boundary."

Dulce muses that she is learning and says,

"I think that Cyan's intentions are much darker. Many of the Wallabies are young and luscious. Some Wallabies are older, fermented and sometimes challenging, and Cyan thinks they are all hers to mould. They all fear Cyan, and they don't trust her. I'm sure that she spends her evenings plotting her plans for their demise for the next day. Cyan toys with them, and she intimidates and wrestles with them. If they come close to winning, she will change the goalposts to a death roll. She has her own rules, and if you break one, she will hurt you. Cyan will chomp you up, spew you out for her Crabs to eat the leftovers and then you will be gone.

If Cyan sees an opportunity for you to assist her, she will generally be charming, pleasant and even seductive in sharing her food and herself. Her Crabs love her. The Crocodile elders only see her charm and conscientiousness as she hurriedly scales up the structural ladder towards them."

Rule number four.

Do not shoot for a goal because Cyan will consistently change the goalposts as the ball leaves your hand so that the ball misses its target.

Do not be solely results-driven. Focus on Cyan's ever-changing detail of detail.

Know that Cyan is always right, and you are always wrong.

If you discover a solution, she will change the goalposts and even do a death roll with you in her clutches. Then she will bury you in the mangroves because you are wrong.

"I can imagine Cyan sitting all alone in her mudslide on the banks of the river, formulating her next intimidation act on the Wallabies. I imagine that the Crocodiles above her keep their distance because she frightens them, but then again, they are just like her, arrogant and opinionated, and they probably frighten her. I have noticed that Cyan can be sugary sweet when she sees that others can assist her needs, and then she can even become seductive and charming," muses Dulce even more," And then there are the rules, those overwhelming rules," sighs Dulce.

Rule number five.

Do as I say and take the full responsibility that I give to you, and then I can, can't I blame you for the train wreck. And I can because this institution employs more like me, who are my line of report. They blame and shame me, and then I release the blame and shame to you, my Wallabies.

Dulce takes the rules seriously and says quietly,

"Looking around, Cyan seems to be in denial that she can see that she is productively producing overwhelming stress in her Wallabies. She seems to be pushing towards her goals for fear of not reaching them and creating stress by pushing her Wallabies too. Cyan doesn't realise that her creation of stress leads to a drop in the wallaby's performance and productivity," Dulce continues to murmur to herself,

"Someone needs to tell Cyan that process is more important than perfectionism because perfectionism is the circle of destruction. Besides, I have read that perfectionism can be a risk factor for obsessive-compulsive disorder. Someone needs to remind her that we are all perfect already in our imperfections. She chases perfectionism and claims to be obsessive-compulsive. I reckon Cyan has obsessive-compulsive disorder. She is consistently obsessive as she successfully creates a lack of motivation that perpetuates a dysfunctional team. I am wondering if Cyan is aware of the chaos that her cunning and manipulation creates. Every word has to be her word, and every punctuation belongs to Cyan. If you dare to change the formatting to meet the institution's rules, you will be chomped up and spat out because you have not formatted according to Cyan's rules."

Dulce stops and shakes her head and then continues,

"She regularly changes all of the goalposts, with no one knowing what to expect next. The Wallabies sit and gossip about her just out of the Crabs' earshot. Gossip comes naturally to them because Cyan is heartless, lacks empathy and fuels the Wallabies talk. Sometimes she pretends to care as she entices her prey into the darkness of her cave, where she can park her prey with their mental health issues of depression and anxiety and then torments them some more."

Dulce and the other Wallabies believe that Cyan is possibly an analytical narcissistic Crocodile, and some believe that she is just a corporate psychopath. Sadly Cyan is Dulce's boss making Dulce a prime target for the energy vampire that Cyan is.

"I'm getting to the point where I breathe deeply to lessen the fear of Cyan that creeps into every nerve ending in my body. I can only think of her as evil, and yet I still try to please her. I remember the time when Cyan's boss caught Cyan out for not performing. Cyan was quick to lay blame and shame at my feet and tormented me in front of my team,"

Dulce sighs and then continues,

"Just like that day when Cyan sidled up to me and asked, "What do you do all day, Dulce? I have no idea?" I remember looking into Cyan's tiny, sad eyes that reflect her small, unhappy and insecure heart. I remember thinking that Cyan thinks strong is intimidation, and creating harmony is about creating discord. Cyan seems to believe that she is a fearless leader, but she isn't because she consistently disempowers, blames and shame. She plays dangerous games with her staff, chomps them up, and spews them out like a Crocodile with indigestion."

Dulce scratches her forearm and sighs and then rants some more,

"Cyan is asking me what I do. If Cyan were here as long as I am each day, she would know because she sits close to me to watch what I do over my shoulder. My productivity probably does fall because I am always wrong, and then I have to redo it and redo it. Cyan consistently waits until I have broken the back of a project before saying that I have to go back to the start."

Dulce stops to scratch her head and then continues,

"If I break Cyan's rules, I know I am in trouble because Cyan will aim her potentially deadly spears of incrimination at me. She likes to breathe her acetone smelling breath at me that primes me for her death roll, and then she watches me tremble until I agree to take the blame for her.

As time passes, it seems that Cyan, the acetone breathing psychopathic narcissist, senses that her empire shows signs of crumbling, and she consistently points the finger at me,"

And as Dulce recalls that she has identified a Cyan weakness, then Dulce smiles and mumbles to herself,

"And as her intimidation and fear tactics rev up, I sense Cyan's panic as she feels that she is losing control of her world out there. Every time she intimidates and incriminates, her Wallabies fall deeper and deeper into despair. They feel even more helpless and hopeless as each day they consistently react to her and then lose their motivation because they are disempowered and threatened. She changes her focus from working towards her end game to look even more closely at each step's precision towards being right because she believes it has worked for her leadership of self and others in the past. It seems that Cyan hides in the depths of detail because it distracts her from making quick decisions. I truly believe that Cyan resembles the Crocodile hiding in the mud at the edge of the mangroves because she hides in the muddy detail of her work. She focuses even more closely on one point at a time, drilling profoundly and even more deeply into each detail as the control of her outer world diminishes even further. The deeper Cyan digs into the detail, and the more unsure her footing becomes and even more unsteady with every step she takes until she appears to be so deep that her supporting side crumbles too, leaving her all alone stuck in the mud. Cyan tries to get unstuck by pivoting in circles. She spins and chomps once, twice, and three times when she decides to empower the Crabs waiting patiently by her side to devour the leftovers. She empowers the Crabs to undermine the Wallabies, and that includes me. The mangroves are thick and isolating, with nowhere for me to run,"

Dulce can feel the tears welling in her eyes, but she just can't stop talking to herself,

"Cyan, the narcissistic, psychopathic Crocodile, lies in wait and observes me many times over, timing her attack to bring me down. Snap, Cyan closes her jaws, chomping me up and spitting me out. Cyan's Crabs lie in wait for their time to clean up the mess. Sometimes Cyan plays with me to tenderise me. Cyan will send me conflicting messages to confuse me by pretending to be my friend. When I least expect it, she will knife me in the back with building rumour, making up barely credible stories about me and sharing them in my professional life out there, bringing my reputation into ill repute.

And as Cyan appeals to my vulnerability and honesty to befriend her, she sets me up to feel weakened and defenceless. That's when my self-doubt builds even more to the point of thinking that I am even more diminutive than not enough. I remember when Cyan set up her laptop computer next to my workstation. She tapped away for a bit and then leant towards me with eyes glowing and her acetone breath distracting me and asked,

"You knew, didn't you?" asks Cyan.

"Knew what?" asks Dulce

"The rumour mongering about a crab and the Wallaby's indiscretion of sharing the rumour." spits Cyan

"Cyan took my breath away, and then I remembered that I kept my head down and continued typing because I knew that Cyan had played her part in a cover-up. One of her Crabs deliberately shared the information with the Wallabies, and it seemed that Cyan wanted to blame and shame me for spreading rumours." Mutters Dulce inside her head.

Then Dulce remembered the rest of the inquisition questions when she said,

"I had heard a rumour."

"Well, why didn't you tell me?" snapped Cyan.

"If I told you about a rumour, then you would have to discipline me for spreading rumours," responded Dulce.

I remember that Cyan turned her head to hide the angry redness creeping into her neck because she knew that I was right, and she had to admit defeat. Cyan didn't admit defeat. She angrily spat out the following words.

"You should have told me never the less."

Dulce stopped for a sip of water and then continued,

"Cyan could discipline me for not reporting the rumour that I heard, or she could punish me for spreading rumours. A lose-lose situation for me. And it was because Cyan recorded her perception of our conversation to my personnel record. Another black mark against me for future reference. And then Cyan disciplined numerous staff for spreading rumours and intimidating others. She delighted in the hurt she caused that grew discontent amongst all her staff. I reckon that Cyan, the psychopathic narcissist, wanted to burn everyone because Cyan burned everything around her and then exalted in laying blame and guilt on me," mumbled Dulce.

And as Dulce absorbed others energy and inadvertently took responsibility for the fault laid on her, she still made excessive efforts to fit in. And as Dulce built pressure within herself, then her world started crumbling around her.

Dulce seeks professional help.

"It is hard work to meet work outcomes when the extent of her communication is, "just do it," is a confusing command. I'm comparatively new to this job, and she's been here long enough to know what she requires me to do. All I ask is a clear framework so that I have certainty of how to move forward," Dulce tells her Counsellor.

"Ask for direction and ask her to specify," responds Dulce's Counsellor.

Dulce thinks about that comment.

"Okay, I will try again to seek clarity, "mutters Dulce.

Dulce thinks about the last time she approached Cyan for direction and clarity and shares her experience with her Counsellor,

"Cyan yells at me and says that I should just know!"

Dulce rubs her left upper arm with her right hand and then continues,

"Cyan holds our weekly meetings for the two of us in the big room where the sound amplifies and bounces around the four walls. I always feel like a trapped animal. I can even feel my eyes widen, my mouth dry, my sweat build, and I know that I sit as still as a frightened animal of prey at every one of her meetings because Cyan watches and waits her time just like a Crocodile. And as she lets Silence fill the room, she will stare at me with glaring intense, darkened eyes that burn through me like a bolt of fire. I am always lost for words, and I do not want to cry in front of her, so I say nothing."

Dulce stops to draw breath, then continues,

"I wonder if Cyan's mother named her that so she can extend her name to Cyanide when she is cross with her," says Dulce.

Dulce fights a smile forming from the corners of her mouth then says,

"She's certainly explosive when you expect and when you least expect it."

Dulce draws another deep breath and continues talking to her Counsellor,

"The targeting consistently continues, and when I think I have done well, Cyan tells me how badly I have done. It seems that everything that goes wrong is my fault, even when it is Cyan's mistake. Cyan is so good at laying blame at my feet when I least expect it. I feel exhausted. I'm not too fond of the place I work in because no matter what I do or how hard I work and give 100% to this institution, it is always wrong. I guess I just need to leave and find another job. I've applied for jobs, and I have been thinking about my options."

"Sounds like you have already decided to leave. It seems to me, and in your mind, you have already left," says the Counsellor.

"Well, I have applied for other jobs. I feel that my applications are flavoured with my feelings of doubt and not feeling good enough. Sometimes I feel like I just spew words onto a page and send that off to prospective employers because I am not successfully gaining an interview," says Dulce.

Dulce stops to breathe and fight back the tears, then she continues,

"Just as well, I have been prescribed old fashioned antidepressants for a temporary severe health issue to help me control the pain. Even though I don't need them for pain now, I do believe that they help me cope with my nasty boss."

Dulce breaks the Silence in the room and continues speaking to her Counsellor,

"Taking antidepressants is more helpful than the advice I have received to hide in an office behind closed doors and lose me in surfing the internet or cry behind the closed toilet door where I remembered the words get over it. More often than not, I remember that behind those doors were posters telling staff that this institution does not tolerate domestic violence. Interesting to note the behaviour that this institution will tolerate in the workplace.

So many times, I would sit and take a nervous pee and feel myself shaking as I stood up and opened the door. I would try to prepare and tell myself that I needed to brace for the next onslaught. Sometimes she would attempt to draw me into her story. I knew that getting off the victim cycle was my way out of her story. I would never know when Cyan would play the victim and share her victim stories with me to feel sorry for her. Sometimes she would be poised for a battle to persecute me through intimidation. Sometimes she would invite me to share a coffee with her to get information about others' behaviour. She would sympathise and then tell me that the other person's behaviour towards me was breaching workplace health and safety, and she would take action to remedy the situation. She never did because it would mean that she would have to discipline her Crabs," says Dulce.

Dulce stops to take a sip of water and then continues,

"If I don't get off the victim cycle, I will experience an even heavier weight of anxiety and depression that will fall on my shoulders.

I think I said too much at the last meeting. I was distracted, thinking that I should not invite Cyan to join me for a picnic in the mangroves where the other Crocodiles live, and their Crabs feed on the other Crocodile's leftovers. This mangrove Crocodile may not be able to digest a whole body of a corporate psychopath because of her hardened attitude. There would be evidence of foul play to explain. I have to think of something else."

Dulce pauses to take a breath before continuing her repertoire. Then she speaks,

"Every time I open the main door of the staff bathroom and step out, I feel the atmosphere around me intensify. I feel the moisture dripping from the palm of my hand as I wipe my sticky fingers down my work pants. I lick my dry lips as I cautiously step back into the world of dreaded expectation. I wait for the bucket full of hellfire and damnation to tip over me."

Dulce's Counsellor sighs and suggests,

"It seems that your workplace problems may lay with Cyan; however, Dulce, you do need to take responsibility for your emotions and behaviour and not give your power to Cyan. Dulce, you need to stop being a people pleaser."

And as Dulce questions her sanity, she flips her questioning and begins to feel better listening to her Counsellor's reassurance. Her Counsellor says,

"Cyan is out of line. Take some time to recover and relax. Exercise and enjoy some time for yourself. Feel free to ring me anytime that you need to," advises Dulce's Counsellor.

Dulce's recovery process is short-lived.

"Hello, it's Dulce here. I need to speak with you. I'm stressing out. That voice in my head is talking over my cacophony of thoughts, telling me not to do anything because I can't do, I can't do anything, so stay safe and don't do anything. I'm listening, and I can't move my feet. I feel stuck out here in the windy weather. I want to cry, but they told me not to let them see me cry. I try to quiet my mind and think of other things, but my internal voice is getting stronger. I feel that I had moved out of the victim cycle, but now I know that I don't know-how. I don't know where to turn. Management brings in a consultant to cut staff and save money, and then the dissatisfied culture drops even further. Productivity drops because people are overwhelmed with so much to do. They procrastinate because they don't know where to begin, and productivity falls to an all-time low. Sick leave increases, people leave or develop health issues, sometimes they develop serious health issues. They bring in a specialist to fix the problem, which means more staff cuts and any sense of security for staff is out the window.

I want to fight, but my strength is waning. I could fly away, but I need another job to fly towards, and right now, I remain stuck in freeze. I'm finding it difficult to catch my breath and engage my brain. I feel like I am stuck here and stuck there. How do I change what is happening to me? How do I change Cyan and her cohorts? I need to stay because I need to earn money. My antidepressants aren't working. Maybe I need to change them and try some that other staff have told me works for them.

I'm in the car park and feel my feet stick to the tarmac as if my shoes are full of lead. I can't make them move."

Dulce's Counsellor listens and waits for Dulce to finish her rant, then says,

"You have returned many times before, and you can do it again. Get over it and move on because you have done it before, and you can do it again. When we finish talking, ring your doctor to make an appointment to discuss your prescription."

"Okay, I will ring my doctor. I can do that."

Dulce's thoughts are racing, and she says,

"I can't do this job. I'm incompetent, and I know this because Cyan tells me every day. Cyan scolds me for having sugar in my coffee because she says that I am unhealthy. I sense that she tells me to do stuff to set me up for failure. I'm beginning to believe it is me, but I need the money. I need antidepressants to help me cope."

Dulce stops to think some more. Dulce's Counsellor has given her the space of Silence, and when Dulce is ready, she continues,

"I have worked in this industry for over 20 years. So if I am not capable, then how have I sustained my work career in this industry?" Dulce sighs heavily and continues,

"I need more help than antidepressants. Even though I believe antidepressants are prescribed to raise serotonin levels because I believe that feeling consistent pain depletes serotonin levels. I have decided that they are helping me, and I believe that they numb my pain. Right now, I feel stuck under a heavy corporate psychopath's weight. That weight undermines my sense of self-confidence and my feeling of self-esteem. I need to feel how I did at previous workplaces. I need to feel valued for the work that I do."

Dulce's Counsellor thinks for a moment and then says,

"I would like to share with you something. I recently read a quote that may resonate with you, Dulce,

Until you heal the wounds of your past, you are going to bleed. You can bandage the bleeding with food, with alcohol, with drugs, with work, with cigarettes, with sex; But eventually, it will all ooze through and stain your life. IyanlaVansant (https://www.goodreads.com/ quotes/101592).

And that's right. You need to find your way to stop the bleeding."

Dulce rubs her left arm with her right hand and then says,

"I think I get it. I understand that I can no longer bandage my bleeding with antidepressants. I can choose to know that I can choose to take the learnings from my past. I know that I can choose to climb that high mountain to take me away and high up. I'm beginning to understand that I need to rise above the many levels of negative emotions and limiting beliefs that I have created and buried deep down below. I have tried to sink them further down by using antidepressants, and for me, I chose to believe that they have helped, but I need more."

At the end of the conversation, Dulce realises that she does know what she has to do. Dulce says goodbye and then mumbles,

"I need to break my pattern of people-pleasing and empower myself to believe in myself. I know that I like variety in my life and like to connect with people, and I now understand that I need to be more selective, and I need to know how to believe in myself. My Counsellor suggested that I need to heal my wounds and take my learnings with me, and then I can take the steps towards planning to step into a new job." Dulce smiles and takes a sip of her water, and then continues,

"I know now that I need to learn how to take responsibility for me and not for Cyan's behaviour."

Dulce continues to smile because she feels like she has hope and has released a weight from her shoulders. A smile relaxes her face muscles and many other muscles in her body. Feeling lighter, she says,

"I have a starting point. I have what I understand, and now I just need to know how."

CHAPTER THREE

Debbie – The force of destruction

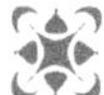

She's courageous.

She taunts and teases and takes her time to blow, destroy until she decides to move on.

Debbie is a strong woman who bends for no one. She is who she is, and Debbie knows what she wants, and Debbie takes what she needs and leaves destruction behind her. Just like the narcissist that she is.

Cyclone Debbie made landfall on the mainland on Tuesday, four hours after prediction.

She lingered and played on the outlying islands moving slowly towards the mainland in her own good time.

Debbie by name and Cyclone by nature,

A stronger woman you could not meet,

Nor would you want to encounter her tantrums and stinging glee,

Her wrath, her taunting, her viscous breaths were pushing, pulling and tearing anything in her way.

Debbie played around, she procrastinated,

She taunted and teased as she hauntingly howled,

She bellowed at the world in her path.

Debbie gave no respite, showed no compassion,

She pushed so hard that corrugated iron sheets thrashed on rooftops,

The screws popped,

The corrugated iron sheets of our safe room smashed against their steel purlins before flying through the air towards their unknown destination.

Her breaths were too strong to fight any longer.

The corrugated iron sheets were flying through the air, across the skies, over rooftops, bouncing on the updrafts, falling with the downdrafts and soaring through the cross drafts.

Sheets of iron creaked as they twisted and turned until they smashed into a tree wrapping around its denuded trunk, protecting that trunk from further torment.

The same tree stood in its glory only hours earlier, with thick green foliage standing tall as it danced in the breeze and sparkled in the sunshine.

Debbie had stolen its leaves every last one, stolen its bark leaving the tree naked and exposed it to the howling winds and blackness around her.

Debbie stole rooftops; she knocked houses from their stumps. She stole windows, doors and security doors, sweeping them up and blowing them many metres into the air and down into the paddocks next door.

She pushed water down through rooves, in through locked windows and up through the cracks where the walls meet the floors.

Debbie cackled, she sneered, she challenged, and she was pushing everything and everyone beyond their limits.

Debbie would make grown men cry.

Then there was the reprieve for one hour or more when the eye of the Cyclone was overhead.

Dogs smiled as they relieved themselves outdoors, birds found refuge in human environs; humans sighed and braced themselves for the next half of the big blow.

Again she blew even more strongly in the opposite direction this time. She played, she lingered, and she procrastinated for another eight hours.

People clung onto front doors challenging Debbie to steal them away.

For eight hours, Echo clung onto the big glass sliding doors opening and shutting them to balance the pressure created by cyclone Debbie.

Debbie blew a window from its frame onto the bed below.

The glass had bowed with the pressure of the wind.

Echo lifted the window and expertly returned it to be seated in its frame.

The winds uprooted and stripped weeds from the soil whilst torrents of rain formed raging rivers around the houses' foundations.

Debbie was doing her best to taunt us as she eerily jeered and hissed as we were winning the battle of the steal. She had got our security doors, but she wasn't going to get our glass sliding doors.

It was then that the little voice inside Echo's head said, "I don't want to die like this. I don't want to die holding onto these glass doors protecting us from the outside turmoil. If the glass shatters and flies through me at 300+ kilometres per hour, I won't be taking another breath."

I was then distracted by the strong winds screaming like a wicked witch who put a spell on the entire universe. The wind's name was Debbie, and she was not going to beat me.

"She was like a corporate psychopath at its best," said Echo with a smirk on her face.

Cyclone Debbie stripped the tree back to the bare trunk and left leafless branches. The tree that had bent and bowed with every strong wind now stood tall, recovered and regrew.

"It was like the tree shed all of its old and stood strong to regrow its bark and leaves with exuberance and abundance," muttered Echo to the world around her,

"I could do that too. I can stand firm in the alpha woman's face, stand my ground, bend and twist with the flow. Then recover, regrow and rejuvenate. If a tree can do so, then I can stand firm in the face of life and work-life balances. If I can back myself in a storm of destruction and survive comparatively unscathed, I can do this anywhere at any time. I can do this in the face of absurdity in the workplace where staffing numbers decrease. Each staff is expected to take responsibility for two or three people and grow productivity. The troops are stressed and pushed over their limits, becoming confused whilst blaming each other for the fall in productivity."

And as Echo shifted her sense of fear and found the power within her to battle Debbie's onslaught, she felt empowered, and her confidence grew exponentially. Echo discovered the experience of strength and courage that allowed her to develop herself abundantly and with vitality. How can she bottle this experience for application in the darkening workplaces out there?

CHAPTER FOUR

Turquoise – Men at work misbehaving

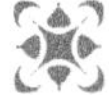

"Beware of the saint, beware of the passive-aggressive charmer. Distinguish between the real and the fake. Focus on deeds and the details of their lives. Focus on how much they seem to enjoy the power and attention, the astonishing degree of wealth they have accumulated, and the number of mistresses, the self-absorption level. Do not become a naïve follower; keep some distance. Enemies shine a light on the hypocrisy," said the podcaster.

"Yes, right," Turquoise says out loud,

"Right now, where I work, men in charge would rather push people around to show hierarchy. The rebels who stood their ground are gone. Now I am in the firing line, and I have symptomatic lower back pain to prove it. I have learned that when my pain increases, my serotonin drops, and as my serotonin drops, my pain increases, which impacts my mental health. Whenever I fear being targeted, I suffer depression because I have flipped into a situation where I sense that I have lost control. I feel redundant and unsupported. I feel the pain of it all in my back, and as I feel my stress level increase, I feel my back pain increase. I mourn what I have lost. Argh, Argh, Argh and other more colourful words is all I can say," says Turquoise,

"I know that Grim and Beastie are mentoring a much younger blue-eyed blonde lady to take my place, and they have directed me to mentor her. Yes, I am older, and Beastie told me that when Grim first met me, Grim said that 'he couldn't get a handle on that woman' and that woman is me, and now I have discovered that they are grooming a much younger staff member to replace me."

Turquoise stops and throws a scrunched piece of paper into the rubbish bin next to her desk. She pushes her auburn hair behind her ears and grimaces, and then Turquoise continues to speak,

"How do they ignore my many successes and many years of experience in this industry that I bring to the table," says Turquoise in between sobs of frustration while trying to make sense of what is happening around her.

Turquoise wipes her eyes with the back of her hand and leaves black mascara streaks down each cheek. She sits in her office with the door closed, talking to her Counsellor on the phone. She takes a sip of hot tea from her favourite delicate china teacup and then says,

"If I go in stronger than my opponents who are trying to push me out of their environment, I might stand a chance. My ego tells me to choose to fight because before the takeover, when I was on the right side of the tracks, I achieved highly and felt my worthiness, and that is where I felt safe. I want to fight for that again, but I will probably have to fight for a severance package instead. The takeover of the institution for whom I worked has changed everything and unsettled everyone, and now the new red-necked patriarchal regime is clumsily pressuring staff from the wrong side of their tracks like me to move on.

Have you heard the term 'getting rid of older ladies past their use-by date?' I wonder if it means restructuring or reorganising in the patriarchal voice?" Turquoise stops and hears her Counsellor say,

"No, I haven't heard that term before."

Turquoise continues,

"I hadn't heard that term either, but now I use that term, 'Getting rid of older ladies past their use-by date' when seeking clarity around its meaning. I asked my bosses whether there were plans to restructure my department as restructuring happens in other departments around me."

"What did they say?" asks Turquoise's Counsellor

"They shook their heads and changed the subject, "Silence falls. Turquoise takes a deep breath, then continues,

"Younger women have replaced a few older women who are much older and older than twenty-five years of age. It seems that all the good staff have left, and here I am," groans Turquoise.

Turquoise's stomach churns, and bile rises into her throat. She senses the weight of helplessness descend on her and into her being. She wants to push her feelings away, but her emotions won't budge. She is stuck. She just sits with them and then builds a story around them.

"Right now, I feel that a dark black emotional mass is descending on me, and now I'm feeling even more afraid."

Turquoise's Counsellor listens and then says,

"Do you know that shellshock and post-traumatic stress can exist on a sliding scale and can affect all of us? Go to your doctor now and ask for stress leave. You are entitled to it."

Turquoise thinks for a moment, and then she responds,

"I have asked my doctor for stress leave, and he pats me on the head and sends me on my way." Turquoise ponders quietly.

Right now, Turquoise just wants to get it all out, and then Turquoise speaks again,

"I have to tell you about Beastie. He's a quiet, smooth-tongued boss who pretends to take the time to listen to his staff. He looks them in the eye. He always smiles and nods at the right time, at appropriate and regular intervals. His team thinks he is industrious when they see him sitting upright in his ergonomically designed desk chair, hiding behind his oversized computer screen. He taps furiously on his keyboard with his end goal in mind, pushing himself to finish his qualification, which will propel him up that corporate ladder that beckons him. Beastie studies diligently towards attaining excellence in task completion to receive recognition from identifying as the person he wants to be.

Now I know that Beastie is a snake in the grass. He shines like a perfect black pearl that would make Captain Jack Sparrow proud, but Beastie strikes like a taipan. One strike and you are dead, all for the common good of eliminating all who present a threat to him. He's a puppet and part of a controlled red-necked cell that hides and governs within a framework of rules, regulations, policies and procedures. Even though the cell's framework is rigid, there's an opportunity to manipulate under the guise of writing procedures that can be re-written to serve his purpose or plan. His squirming slimy body couldn't lie straight in bed even with a rod inserted. A taxidermist would have to compromise and find a crooked rod to stuff dear Beastie. His mind, consumed by his ego, seizes the opportunity to meld the procedures to suit his cause."

Turquoise's Counsellor gives her space to process her thoughts, and after the Silence, Turquoise continues her rant,

"I reckon that Beastie is a multi-personality skilled beast. He lacks empathy for his staff though he knows how to manipulate people, and he lets the people above him manipulate him. He lets them because he wants to be significant to them. He finds it easy to please those more powerful than he is because he wants to be important to them. I can imagine that if the opportunity arose to test his loyalty, he would go so far as tampering with electoral ballot boxes under instruction to please his mentors, of course. And it seems to me that his sponsors are enabling him to climb the corporate ladder quite quickly. Beastie appears to be kind and sincere, but he is unkind and devious. His skill to morph from being lathered in a silky amenable coating to become someone else with an intent to slowly release a poison that will perplex one's mind and drive one into the dark side is unprecedented.

Beware the stronger vulnerable who dares to entertain a different thought. Bam, you are dead or excommunicated. No feelings for the hurt he causes or the poverty he induces because you don't conform to making life easy for him."

Turquoise wipes her eyes with the back of her hand and laments the friendship that was.

"Once we were friends, or so I thought. Now Beastie just questions me."

"Do you go home and kick the dog because of the way we are treating you?" Beastie asks me whilst he smiles smugly."

"And how do you respond?" asks Turquoise's Counsellor

"I always say no because I love dogs." Turquoise then says,

"I remember when Beastie said,

"considering the previous life traumas that you have survived, you will easily be able to survive what we're doing to you now."

I believe that Beastie watches me closely because he waits for the cracks in my emotions to appear. Then he strikes, or he pokes me a little more in the hope of generating a reaction. And then he fires even more of his questions at me,

"Well, your husband would be supportive, wouldn't he?"

I remember Beastie's smirks and how he almost drooled with enjoyment. He is so wrong to speak to me like that," says Turquoise. She stops to take in three deep breaths and then continues her rant,

"Beastie acts as though he believes that he's always right because he's protected, and that is his reward. He lives up there on that high pedestal of rightness. His rightness is reinforced up the corporate ladder with his big boss, Slippery Jim being Beastie's second supporter after Grim."

Turquoise blinks the tears from her eyes and breathes deeply to change the focus of her thoughts, and then says,

"I reckon that the chase for well-presented women stirs Grim, who clumsily flirts and then fights off the desire to transgress a second time because he's decided to immerse himself in loyalty for his current wife? Forever loyal to the one he keeps at home barefoot and pregnant.

Slippery Jim is cheered by his Bouncy Sidekick, who is young with an energetic body. She brings a smile to his face daily, and then he encourages her to beat the troops. God help those who think for themselves. Bouncy Sidekick bullies the staff with slippery Jim's blessing. Humiliation is the key, she thinks, but it is quite funny to watch her wiggle her finger, yell like a machine gun spitting out bullets with no time between to defend the preconceived guilty verdict. If you do defend yourself, they will deem that you are even more culpable because you dare to think outside the red square."

Turquoise wriggles in her seat and crosses her arms to contain her anger, and then continues,

"Grim's metaphoric speak, "getting rid of older ladies past their use-by date ", is not about a restructure at all. It is literal about getting rid of whom he is speaking to now. It's all about the fit. If you are young and sexy, you are in like Flynn.

Just like a new broom sweeps clean, new leadership in the dominating takeover institution may brush away the old to make the younger, prettier, compliant new. Sweep out of the older, less vulnerable to replace with a younger, more attractive and compliant model is Grim and Beastie's puppeteers' directive."

Turquoise stops to sip her water and take some time to sort through her thoughts.

Turquoise feels like she is fighting an internal battle,

"I want to stay and feel valued, but I know that's not going to happen, so I think I need to lead myself with the intent of leaving on my terms."

Turquoise's Counsellor nods and suggests,

"I believe that you are beginning to understand and adapt to Beastie's turn from friend to foe."

Turquoise nods in agreeance and then murmurs,

"My friendship with Beastie is dipping deeper and deeper into the red because he has learned to morph into a narcissistic overlord whilst sitting at his desk in front of his oversized computer screen. For him, it was right for him to step away from friendship to be the narcissistic overlord, and he does it well," sighs Turquoise loudly and stops to think. Tears well in her eyes, and she chews her bottom lip whilst searching for answers on the wall in front of her. Then Turquoise continues,

"I remember another time not so far back when my best friend and partner turned from friend to foe in what seemed like a moment that stopped time. I arrived home from a scuba diving weekend earlier than planned. I was tired, hungry, and filled with excited anticipation to share my adventure stories of the last two days with my most trusted and loyal l friend and then partner, Golly.

I could hardly contain my excitement as I recalled how exciting it was to swim with majestic stingrays, collect scurrying scallops on the seabed. We ate the delectable scallop delicacies on a pizza prepared later that evening, and generally, I had lots of fun. Golly had encouraged me to learn to scuba dive, and I did it successfully. I wanted to share my wins and my appreciation with Golly," Turquoise says and then breathes deeply.

"I remember telling myself that Golly will be so proud of me and will want me to share my adventures. I believed that I was so lucky to share successes with Golly because we were best friends, and I knew that he loved me. Then as I walked towards the door, I could hear the sound of soft music beckoning me. I walked through the door into the kitchen and saw what I saw. Golly was sitting at the kitchen bench with a friend, my best girlfriend, Lincoln. I remember thinking that they would be just as excited as me to listen to my stories. I walked towards them with the intent of sitting with them when something stopped me. My mouth fell open. No sound emerged. I watched the oyster topped savoury biscuit being offered and placed into Lincoln's mouth. I could feel saliva build in my mouth, and I licked my lips. I watched Lincoln smile appreciatively as she received the succulent morsel from Golly, who was sitting beside her. The more I concentrated on their actions, the more I could feel myself going into the trauma of being stuck in confusion. I tried to move my legs, but I was stuck on the one spot watching them. That's when I realised that they had just noticed me because they quickly looked away. It was then I realised that my best friend Lincoln had betrayed me. I watched Lincoln as she focused on Golly's face as she slowly savoured the sensual morsel in her mouth. They were sitting at my kitchen bench with a spread of oysters, my favourite oysters that I had bought in my last shop. Savoury biscuits were spread on the plate in the middle of the bench, with wine-filled crystal glasses sitting in front of them. I felt like my mind froze, and then my tears fell, and thoughts upon thoughts multiplied in my mind. I felt sick to my stomach. I was shocked. I remember thinking that Golly didn't sit with me like that. Golly is my partner, a friend and confidante, the one I trust most in this world. My best friend, Lincoln, how could she? So many thoughts. They were colliding in my mind. Golly was initially excited about doing a scuba diving course, and then he pulled out at the eleventh hour. I knew that Golly must be curious about my scuba diving adventures. Golly told me that Scuba diving is one of the best things and would be one of the best things to happen in our lives. Golly was initially going to do it with me. Then I remembered that I had forgotten to remember that Golly had pulled out of the scuba diving experience at the eleventh hour. Now I remember that Golly had substantially increased my life insurance at the same time. My head was spinning, so I took a deep breath, looked up towards the ceiling and then looked back at them. That's when I remembered feeling like my head was going to explode, I could hear my stomach rumble and churn, and I could feel my throat constricting as each breath became shallower. Golly and Lincoln only had eyes for each other, and I was invisible to them,"

Turquoise wipes the tears from her cheeks and reaches for a tissue to blow her nose, and then continues,

"I had always welcomed Lincoln and her family into my home, and then she did this to me. I didn't know whether I should be angry or cry. I remember feeling numb, confused and stuck because it quickly became clear that everything right now indicated that I could not trust anything that these two said, did, or described. Golly had criticised me for being too trusting of people, and these were the people I couldn't trust. I couldn't believe that my then-partner thought my best friend was worth more to him than me."

Turquoise groans and fiddles with her when she finds her voice to say,

"The world is a difficult place to be. I can only feel how hard life is because of what people are doing to me. They're excluding me when I don't conform and making me feel rejected. You know that horrible feeling of not being good enough. The further into my life's journey that I embark, I discover more and more my belief intensify that I am not good enough, and I can feel my fear of being found out that I'm not good enough grow even more."

Silence falls as she thinks some more. Turquoise's Counsellor encourages Turquoise to continue,

"What else have you learned?"

"I have learned to know the flavour of adventure that motivates me to fight for what I desire. A generous payout is my desire, or maybe I will settle for leaving when I have secured another job a long way away from here. There is part of me who wants to stay and a part of me that wants to run. So if both my parts wish the best for me, then what? I guess I would need to be flexible, and whenever I'm unsure of what part to listen to, I can seek clarity through my journaling."

Turquoise wrinkles her brow, bites her bottom lip, and then says,

"I remember that day not long after the takeover when Grim began his tyranny of publicly humiliated me in front of my staff. I remember my anger expanding in my chest, and I decided to say nothing. Instead of waiting until the end of the meeting, I hid in my office. A place where I could hide behind my computer screen and journal. I remember that it was only days into the new regime, or so it seemed, when I realised what I had lost. They crippled and stripped me of any opportunity for achieving highly. Now my sense of worthiness lies in my past. A pre-takeover manager warned me to run, and I ignored this warning. I remember I just wanted to cry. If I cried, I knew that Grim and Beastie would be encouraged to go in harder. So I chose to use my tea break to smash out my journaling, and I wrote this little gem.

Grim and Beastie went to war.

Grim got squashed by an apple core.

No, it wasn't. It was a rock.

Beep beep beep flies past at sixty miles per hour.

He just didn't run fast enough.

Oh, you didn't mean that he runs.

He works as he runs

Yes, that would be right.

He runs so fast he doesn't even take the time to listen.

He micromanages, humiliates and whips those he pays to serve him.

Sniff, sniff, sniff…" oh, it's dark in here," says Beastie quietly, not wanting to ruffle any fur, "It burns in here. It must be gastric juices?"

Sit you brutes and stay.

The heads pop out of their kennels tentatively, searching for instructions.

The chains around their necks are pulled so tight,
So tight to stop the flow of their intelligence fluid
That intelligence fluid so needed to lubricate the thinking source.
Tentatively they take a step, watching for approval.
The approval nod and the tales wag
Wag in unison with relief that another beating is yet postponed.
Beastie's almost hidden.
Is it Grim's tail we can see wagging, or is it Beastie's legs we can see flapping?
Wack the scythe is falling quickly everybody run
Run fast, back into your kennels."

Turquoise's Counsellor sits quietly and observes Turquoise, and then Turquoise begins to speak some more,

"I used to wonder when the honeymoon would end, and then the takeover happened, and boom, the honeymoon was over, and then I find myself smashing the keys on the keyboard journaling and writing this stuff."

"What do you mean by honeymoon?" asks Turquoise's Counsellor

"The calm and harmonious period where I moved forward to achieve success. I celebrated successes and felt supported by the people I worked for, and the people I worked with that is the six years before the takeover," says Turquoise.

Turquoise fiddles with her hair and wipes the tears in her eyes. She feels angry and sad and just wants to find her happiness once again. Turquoise continues her rant,

"Grim and Beastie go to great lengths to dissuade me from staying. They consistently humiliate me in front of my team and ensure that every meeting with me includes my team. They continuously decrease my authority and increase my responsibility in my position, and they do this in front of everyone. Not only did I release my emotions by writing poems, journaling, or making up stories, I would often wonder, does Beastie load the gun for Grim, or do they lock and load each other's gun, and that is the question?

The tips of their heads are brown with frantic rubbing causing baldness. I wonder, what are they doing to cause blindness, but they can see, can't they?

Slippery Jim's coat is brown, that dry, flaky brown that comes from sliding up and down that dark, dirty hole where he hides and flickers into light when so told. Big Red is the newly appointed King and puppeteer of the newly formed institution."

Turquoise ponders her childish thoughts that make her smile, and then she remembers,

"I'm not the only childish one because so important was Big Red that Someone wrote an ode.

An ode to Big Red

There was a place named Flowin.
Who joined with another place they said was owin'?
So they proceeded to rape, plunder and pillage
The tithes increased, and there was spillage.
Big Red promised to seal the Pongo dirt Road.

> But alas, this section was an Engineers ode.
> To build and maintain a bitumen road.
> Across this section of unmade road
> An engineer's nightmare, it would be
> To stop the waters of the rising sea.
> Big Red's nightmare it would be.
> His coffers are decreasing, he would see.
> The fortune he saw amassing for a run at pre-selection
> Within the newly formed boundaries for this election
> Big Red made many a promise.
> But he turned out to be a lying poly redneck prick.
> Staff left in droves from the place that was owin' because Big-Red
> gave jobs to his boys from Flowin."

Turquoise is on a roll because she hurts so much and continues her rant,

"I decided that I like to think of Big-Red's face looking washed out because he needs to come up for air. His unspoken mantra is if you comply, you will have security in my workplace. He lacks compassion, and other peoples' lives mean little to him. If you dare to disagree with him, he will hurt you. Turn your back, and he will hunt you down, and he will not hesitate to knife you in your back, and he too will dump you lifeless and heavy into the jaws of the waiting crocodile whose crabs patiently wait to demolish the leftovers. No evidence is left behind and, therefore, no recriminations. And that is the norms of his individuals' and his institution's behaviour that is his cultural creation.

Under the covers, he jumps with each young lass feeling special and the next feeling even more special only to find that they were not the one but one of many. These younger women were ripe for the picking. The older men's smiles and compliments were like a magnet to these young girls. They loved to hear how special they were. They felt the feel-good emotions race within them. The attention meant job security too but only for as long as they were desirable and compliant."

Turquoise winces as she shares her elaborate stories with her Counsellor. Turquoise thinks for a moment, takes a sip of water, then continues,

"I remember that night when the older men lured young women to party time with the call of copious amounts of free alcohol. It was a party that Big Red threw for all staff, and I felt obliged to attend. My staff were smarter than me, and they declined his invitation. My observations overwhelmed me, and I witnessed more than my job description required. I ate my free finger food and drank my free drink, and then I left the building. I later heard that the alcohol was flowing as much as you could drink and more. Big Red and his cohorts called a taxi to take their wives home so that they could be free to stay and play. When I heard how the alcohol flow primed the young women, I heard that some of these young women were falling over, and one fell into the gutter. The emancipated husbands helped them up because they were ready to play. I realised then that I had heard enough, and I was glad that I didn't wait to see."

Turquoise stops to breathe and take a sip of her water,

"Sooner or later, I will know how to resolve this change in my work-life because I will flee this institution sooner or later because I don't understand its culture. The post takeover culture is the exact opposite of what it was.

I can only perform as requested and as well as I can to meet my contract agreement. And now, my immediate boss expects me to drag my work backwards to his pre takeover level, and then he will randomly set the bar much higher than it has ever been for him. Nothing I do meets with approval. So I have begun to do more of nothing. They have let me know that I am an old lady past her use-by date, so what do I have to lose? I'm only here treading water until something better comes along."

Turquoise stops to think and screws up her face as she realises she is becoming like them. She mumbles,

"I feel like I am compromising my value of integrity which doesn't sit well with me. My desire to leave on my terms is becoming even more significant and pressing."

Turquoise shakes her head as though she were shaking the guilt from her, and then she justifies,

"I remember hearing that we are the average of the people with whom we spend the most time. I spend most of my waking hours with these people, so it's not my fault that I waste work time as they do. Beastie wastes time tapping out his papers for assessment, and Grim wastes time running around like the roadrunner. Grim moves quickly but progresses slowly with his micromanaging work methods. So they are getting what they are giving. I think I have made up good excuses."

Turquoise takes a big sip of water and then continues,

"You know I requested clarification around getting rid of older women past their use-by date. I asked my bosses, and they ignored me, so then I put my request in writing, and this is what I wrote,

Dear Grim,

You mentioned that Slippery Jim was getting rid of older ladies past their use-by date, and I wondered if that meant you were changing our workflows or even restructuring our area?

I am just seeking clarification for our business plan.

Yours sincerely, Turquoise."

"What happened then?" asks Turquoise's Counsellor.

"I got a response almost immediately. A furious Grim appeared at my door and proceeded to haul me across the coals for spreading rumours. Then he organised a meeting with Bouncy Sidekick for the three of us to attend. He told me he wanted to meet to discuss operational matters. It turns out I was their operational matter because I had asked about restructuring.

I didn't have a chance to speak in the meeting with Grim and Bouncy Sidekick firing their words at me with the speed of machine-gun fire, so I thought it seemed real to me that they were planning a restructure that wasn't a restructure."

Turquoise sips her water and then says,

"The possibility of a restructure was fuelled in my imagination by fear, or was it? I noticed the there were already major changes happening with older ladies leaving. The institution was quick to recruit younger women to fill many vacant positions, which meant that the institution needed to hire casuals to fill the post-school hours of the day. When the younger women were unavailable, Slippery Jim wanted us to believe that the younger women had to take time off to make their school runs and weren't available for the last hours of the day. That was a massive change to the structure. ?"

"And then what happened?" Turquoise's Counsellor asks Turquoise,

"Our meeting ended when the machine-gun fire of words, incriminations and finger-wagging stopped. It was then that I knew that I had to leave, but there was still a flicker of determination to stay until I could go on my terms.

"How did you feel when you left the meeting?" Turquoise's Counsellor asks Turquoise,

Turquoise sighs heavily and continues to speak,

"I felt like I was immersed in a black shadow of nothingness, and I felt like I was drowning in pain and irritants. My back hurt, and my allergies increased because I felt unsupported and I felt unsafe. My intent for staying, or so I told myself, was to leave on my terms, and that would be when I have another job to go to," Turquoise tells her Counsellor.

Turquoise stops talking and observes the thoughts hurtling through her mind. Right now, in this place, equality of the sexes, are you kidding me. It seems to me that in this environment, the patriarchal white supremacists hold power and are motivated by their brains' blood flow into that part of them that leads them to transgress. I feel like I am in a time warp. I guess that's a bit harsh, but it is my truth as I see my world."

Turquoise stops to catch her breath, then says,

"Why is it that when women demonstrate their dominant strength, they are called bitches, but when men show their dominance, they identify as strong. Interesting! You know, I think that Big Red's boys are even more than interesting because, in my mind, they fall under the bad leader brand."

Turquoise's Counsellor asks, "What makes you say that?"

Turquoises' Counsellor allows space for Turquoise to immerse in her thoughts, then listens as Turquoise continues,

"I remember that I had heard about bad leaders and how they are self-absorbed and pretend to be at the centre of every decision. They dictate and create a culture of fear to create chaos and confusion. Bad leaders cannot empower people and fall short on commitment because there is no vision and no clear lines of accountability. They can talk the talk but do not walk the walk. Management will eventually sense bad leaders untruths, and the bad leaders will find themselves marching out. When the bad leaders' sponsors leave, then they do too. And I say that they can take their bullying with them. Could it happen again this time?. It's all about them, and there is a lot of them right now. One day they will be escorted out, and I will hear that they elected to leave, but that day is not today."

Turquoise's Counsellor thinks for a moment whilst playing with her pen, then she says,

"Be careful of the bully who will intimidate you and your team because he will sully your reputation and sing it from the rooftops. He will make it difficult for you to stay and difficult for you to get another job in the same industry if he so wishes. Be very careful that you do not stain your reputation because these bullies will black mark you in your industry."

Turquoise ponders her response,

"Yes, you are right. I need to learn how to work in this environment without compromising my values even further, and then I need to leave,"

Turquoise hesitates before continuing,

"If I remind myself of my achievements, then perhaps I will feel even more valued, inspired and motivated as I have before. I can focus on my values to change my thinking and how I feel now, and then I could take my feelings forward into a new workplace where my achievements would be valued and acknowledged. I have a dream that I will work for an institution whose values mirror mine and a place where I would be treated with respect, appreciation and gratitude once more," says Turquoise in a dreamlike state."

Turquoise's Counsellor acknowledges Turquoise's realisation and says,

"Awesome work Turquoise.".

Destiny – You get what you focus on, so focus on what you want

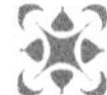

Change your focus to change the meaning of your life's events to choose your choice for your life's changes, because, **The thoughts we think and the words we speak create our experiences – Louise L. Hay** (www.goodreads. com/quotes/7632435)

Destiny found her trusted guide and inspirational mentor in Alice. Right now, Alice is holding space for Destiny. She listens to Destiny, giving her a judgement-free zone to speak her truth to identify her challenges and discover her solutions.

Following the space of silence and partway through the follow on conversation, Alice asks,

"Destiny, is it okay if I share with you?"

"Yes, of course," responds Destiny.

Alice says,

"Our thoughts create our feelings, and not every one of them is precise. Most of the negative emotions like overwhelm, stuck, fear, and doubt should be challenged unless we face the danger of a Crocodile spying on us, and then we would run fast before we became the Crocodile's dinner. If I see a real Crocodile on the river bank with jaws wide open, ready to snap, then I can make it mean that the Crocodile may be a threat. I can face my fear and choose to stay and find out or face my fear and run away towards safety.

Suppose I see a Crocodile picture, and it triggers fear. In that case, I can choose to change that fearful feeling if I change my perspective from the drama of knowing that it is my imaginary truth. I can interpret the picture as a fearsome image and feel the fear, or I can choose to see the actual truth that it is only a picture on a piece of paper. I can decide to make the negative, fearful feeling go away, making space to feel the more resourceful feelings of joy, appreciation, love and gratitude. I can then be grateful that the Crocodile that I see is just a picture."

Destiny thinks for a moment before responding,

"Yes, I get what you are saying. My issue is much larger than changing my thoughts around a picture. I feel that I'm swimming towards a lifebuoy ring that moves further away from me with each of my swimming strokes, making my rescue further away and then out of reach. The more I struggle, the further away my rescue is pushed. So it's time to move again," sighs Destiny and continues,

"I have four weeks to pack up my house and move 1,000 kilometres from here to be in time to start my new job. I am leaving my fear of persecution in the workplace that I am leaving behind." Destiny rubs her face then says,

"I know that I can move away and leave behind the mental anguish." Destiny sighs loudly and continues,

"I found in doing my research that workplace bullying is a significant issue in Australia and many countries worldwide. I discovered that victims or witnesses of bullying have a higher rate of depression, chronic stress leading to mental and physical illnesses, sometimes considering suicide, and I don't want that for me,"

Destiny stops to take a deep breath before continuing,

"In hindsight, I remember feeling depressed a lot. I remember that feeling of a heavy dark veil descending on me, and it would fall without warning. I believe others felt the same because every day, at least one person from my team called in sick. More than half were actively looking for other jobs, and their enthusiasm in their present position waned. Some staff became masters at looking busy but producing very little. I have to get away before these negative emotions set firmly in my system,"

Destiny sighs loudly and breathes deeply, and then continues,

"Last time I ran, I took what I needed in my car, leaving everything else behind me."

Rubbing the side of her face, Destiny falls silent, allowing space for contemplation.

Then Destiny mumbles,

"I found that the more times I ran away from my fears, the more triggers I amassed. It is like feelings of guilt, humiliation and anger cloud around me and wraps me in a dense, heavy greyness that creeps into me from somewhere deep below or falls on top of me from above, sometimes when I least expect it."

Destiny takes three deep breaths and then says,

"I have to get away and leave it all behind me, and that is why I am leaving."

Destiny stops her dialogue and looks up towards the left-hand corner of the room. She gives herself space to think, and then she lowers her eyes and says,

"When my emotions overwhelm me, I don't think that I have the stability to choose to change my thoughts in the midst of overwhelm. I feel a strong drive where I have to get away."

Destiny stops to collect her thoughts and remembers the day she stayed.

"I'll just race over to the fresh fruit and vegetable section because I forgot the pumpkin," she said to her partner, who waited by the shopping trolley.

Destiny remembered leaning across the stuffed shelves to grab a piece of pumpkin when her foot slipped from underneath her. She watched the shelves turn sideways, she held her breath and then she fell heavily. Lying on the cold hard vinyl floor looking up at the legs around her made her think how vulnerable and humiliated she felt. Destiny was upright in two seconds flat. She could feel the parts of her that hurt.

"I can move my legs, and my arms move. My head hurts a bit because it hit the floor heavily when I slipped. I can see clearly. There's no double vision, so all good," she mumbles,

"And I have answered questions for the incident report, so all good."

Destiny stood upright and brushed herself down.

"I'm fine," she said and continued her shopping. She pretended all was well and that her fall never happened.

She rounded the corner into the second aisle, and one of the bystanders was walking towards her.

"Are you okay?" she asked.

Destiny looked at the floor and said,

"Yes, I think so,"

Destiny could feel her neck redden and sensed that negative feeling trigger,

"I feel so embarrassed," whispered Destiny.

"Embarrassed. I would be feeling outraged. To think that the floor was slippery and unsafe."

Destiny turns to Alice and says,

"I remember feeling judged and then guilty for not being angry as I expected, and then I remember my embarrassment intensify. I felt vulnerable and wanted to run from the shop and drive away, but I didn't have the car keys, my partner did, and he didn't want to run.

I remember that my vulnerability triggered my thoughts which would scramble in my mind making me feel embarrassed. I tried to physically move to hide from other people because I feared their judgment. I realised that it is essential to know what other people think of me because I wanted people to like me at that point in my life."

Destiny sips her water and takes time to catch her breath.

"In the scheme of things, it was only a squashed grape that someone had dropped on the floor that had caused me to slip, and total strangers came to help me. So why did I feel like I needed to bow my head and hide behind other shoppers pushing their trolleys? I can still feel that sense of relief when we had finished our shopping. I remember seeing the exit door with the promise of escape loom in front of me. That's when I quickened my step and moved away through the exit towards the safety of anonymity, where I could cry with no one to watch me," Destiny tells Alice.

"How did your feelings change when you reached the place of anonymity?" asks Alice.

Destiny thinks for a moment and then responds,

"I still felt embarrassed, vulnerable, and I could feel a heaviness in my chest, but I felt like I was more in control to choose my place to cry. I still felt embarrassed to the point of not wanting to go back into the store because people may recognise me and judge me. When I think about it, I think that I was afraid that they might think that I am not as good as them."

Alice sits quietly and thinks for a moment.

"Destiny, is it okay if I comment?" Destiny nods and says,

"Yes, please."

"It seems that you are reacting to other people's opinion of you instead of valuing your own opinion of you. You then seem to make the event bigger and bigger. Much bigger than it needs to be. It may be that your opinion of you is where your power lies," explains Alice.

Destiny looks down towards her feet and thinks for a moment, then asks,

"Okay. How do I do that?"

Alice responds,

"My mother would tell me that you need to stop making mountains out of molehills. You will then find that you can more easily manage the smaller chunks of embarrassing events that happen to you. When an awkward moment happens, she would tell me to stop momentarily, take a deep breath and think about my response.

And as you change your thoughts that change your emotions to feel how you choose to feel, you can decide how you choose to think about yourself.

My mother would also tell me to choose to be the magic in my world where I would love myself, and then that love would transfer to others."

Alice stops to give Destiny time to think.

"Is it okay if I share with you what else I have noticed?" asks Alice.

Destiny nods and then listens to Alice,

"I remember you telling me that when life drives you to run, you often feel physical pain in your back and experience anxiety around not feeling good enough that makes your pain worse, and so it continues?"

That's right, "responds Destiny.

Alice continues,

"I am wondering when your feeling of not being good enough triggers your anxiety, and that then you feel overwhelmed, which leads to procrastination. I sense that you have a drop in your productivity at work. When that happens over some time, it seems that it then affects your health. Tell me, how does that serve you?"

There were moments of silence before Destiny responds,

"Well, if my back hurts, then I can get a medical certificate to take sick days. I then have time to recuperate and recover. I get to stay home for as long as I need, watch television or read or sleep. I always feel more robust for my return to face the intimidation attacks and other people's scrutiny of me and my work because then it takes longer to trigger my fear of not being enough. Because I seem to have a reserve of energy."

"If your health deteriorates even further, to the point of you being disabled and suffering chronic pain, how will that serve you?" asks Alice.

Destiny falls silent and then says,

"I won't be able to work, and I will have to rely on others to help me. I will lose my independence and the strength to pursue my interests."

"And how will that serve you?" asks Alice.

Destiny contorts her face muscles and falls into a contemplative silence.

"I don't want to go there," whimpers Destiny.

"What will you choose instead?" asks Alice, allowing Destiny space to think.

Destiny thinks for some time and then remembers a quote that resonates with her, triggering her thoughts.

Though no one can go back and make a brand new start, anyone can start from now and create a brand new ending. – Carl Brand. (<u>https://tinybuddha.com/wisdom-quotes/</u>)

Destiny can feel a smile happening, and she continues speaking,

"I remember reading that if I change my focus, I can change the meaning that I give to my feelings which create how I emote to the world around me. So if I changed my focus in the supermarket to think that I could choose my response to honour me by appreciating that I was okay and grateful, I could happily continue to shop. I would then focus on feeling the excited anticipation to have dinner guests later that day.

So if I change my focus now to choose a different meaning for my life's events, then I can choose the courage to stop to take a moment for me to take a deep breath. I can think good thoughts and then feel good with my response to my life's challenges. I can effectively permit myself to design my desired significant outcome. I can support myself to take baby steps towards my desired outcome, knowing that I can find the courage within to overcome the bumps in the road that I have chosen," says Destiny and then asks,

"Is it that simple to choose my choice for my change?"

"Changing your focus to choose differently is an excellent step," says Alice.

Silence falls, and Alice sits and observes.

"What else would you need to know?" asks Alice.

Alice waits patiently whilst observing Destiny process her thoughts. Destiny appears to recall information from her collection of learnings when she says,

"In my current workplace, I find that everyone is pretending to be my friend when I see them, and then they create ugly gossip whilst laughing at their perceptions of my incompetence to take the focus from their incompetencies or something like that. Even though I know it is just malicious gossip, I feel like I'm missing my fundamental value around connection, which I make mean that my highest value of integrity is compromised."

"What if you could change your focus from what you hear out there and how others colour your world to relying on listening to your internal feedback to appreciate you and understand how you can be who you choose to be to choose how you colour your world ?" asks Alice.

Alice gives Destiny time to think and then listens to Destiny's response,

"That would be awesome."

Destiny sighs and listens to Alice, who shifts from mentor to teacher.

"Let me tell you about a five-step program called **FOCUS** where you can learn to change your thoughts to honour yourself. You can learn to know how to go from feeling disempowered, scared & overwhelmed in a toxic working environment to choosing your choice for your change. You may learn to be the architect of your life and empower yourself to make your life easier in a toxic work environment. You can learn how to choose your change to empower you in your life's journey and be the Architect of your life, or you can learn how to give up what you think the past could have been and free yourself to have a clean now and future even if you believe that you are at the point of giving up."

Destiny thinks for some time and asks,

"Alice, can please you tell me more about your FOCUS program."

Alice says,

"The FOCUS program allows you to discover how you can change your focus to choose your choice for your change.

Step one is Focus and forgiveness - Change your focus and use forgiveness to give up what you think the past could have been. You can change your beliefs to form beliefs that will serve you now and in your future and free yourself to have a clean now and future.

Step two is Opportunity and Possibilities – Change your focus to take up the opportunity to know that all possibilities are available to you now.

Step three is Courage – Change your focus to understand that you have the courage you need within in and you can use courage to influence your choice for your change

Step four is Understanding - Change your focus and use understanding to know that you can make changes at an unconscious level to change at a conscious level to change your life

Step five is Self-talk, synchronise and strategise – Change your focus to support you as you would your best friend and use self talk to build your certainty in self-belief and self - love so that you can master your mind.

What do you think?"

Destiny nods and thinks about Alice's information and then asks,

"Alice, can you elaborate even more, please?"

"Certainly," says Alice and then shows Destiny the Framework for her FOCUS program.

FOCUS

F ocus and forgiveness	Focus on forgiveness to change your beliefs to change your feelings to set you free to make informed decisions to choose your choice for your change. Give up what you think the past could have been and free yourself to have a clean now and future. Focus on what you have now and Focus on what you have in the future. Focus on Gratitude for now. Focus on a healthy outlook for what your future can be.

O pportunity and Possibilities	Quantum physics says that we are the past, the future, and endless moments of now, and all possibilities are available to everyone, which means that they are available to you. Focus on the endless opportunities and possibilities available to you now and in the future and know what they mean to know what action to take. Keep choosing until you find opportunities and possibilities that work for you. Create your SMART goals that create meaning in your life's experiences. Permit yourself to take baby steps towards your desired outcome. If you believe it will work out, you will see opportunities. If you believe it won't, you will see obstacles.- Wayne Dyer (https://www.facebook.com/groups/WayneDyerQuotes)
C ourage	Have the courage to: see what works; eliminate what doesn't work; know that you can create something different as many times as you need to until your life choices align with your values, your purpose and the outcome of your chosen design. Immerse yourself in the current moment to heighten your awareness of what works for you and what you can influence for you. If a boss, an institution or even a town has values and beliefs that contradict yours, then you cannot influence change. If their sense of right is your sense of wrong, you cannot fit or change your external environment. You can choose your choice for your change from all the opportunities and possibilities available to you. You can have the courage to make a clean break where you leave and cut your ties. Just know that carrying the pain with you happens for as long as you remember, reflect and immerse in your painful experiences. Have the courage to let them go as they are not with you in the now or current moment. Have the courage to let go of what doesn't work for you to make space for what works and what you can bring into your life that is new. Have the courage to break habits that do not serve you and know that they are from your historical past. Have the courage to change your behaviour to make new habits that align with your values and purpose.
U nderstanding	Understand that the changes you make to your thinking that creates your emotions happen in the current moment. Understand that you can make changes at an unconscious level to change at a conscious level to change your life even more efficiently and be the person that you choose to be. Understand the behavioural flexibility that enables you to go with the ebbs and flows of your life. You can choose your choice for your change and know that you can adapt as needed.

	Understand that with Hypnotherapy and NLP techniques guidance, you can make changes at an unconscious level to change at a conscious level. And as you change your thoughts that change your feelings, you can change your behaviour to influence your life's experiences. You can be the architect of your life experiences and decide to be flexible to ride the ebbs and flows right now and in your future.
S elf-talk, self-love, synchronise and strategise	Focus on your self-talk. Build your certainty in self-belief for building self-love so that you can master your mind. When you master your mind, amazing things happen. And as you strategise, I know that you can be the architect of your life's experience and design the life of your dreams now, and it is more or less the right thing to do for your future. That means that you will appreciate what you have now. Synchronise your life's experiences with your values to master your mind, change your thoughts to change your feelings, be who you choose to be, do what you can do, and have the feelings you choose to maintain a positive attitude from now on. Develop an awareness of the words you use, be aware of your language, and use it to support you.

"That sounds awesome," says Destiny. She sits with a wrinkled brow as she ponders the FOCUS program information.

Alice smiles and then asks,

"If it is okay with you, I will go through the steps in a little more detail for you."

Destiny nods and makes herself comfortable to listen and learn some more.

Forgiveness - the first step

"Forgiveness is the first step to changing Focus for you to become the best version of you to choose your chosen change choice.

If you take 100% responsibility for your life, back yourself, and forgive your past whilst releasing your resentments, then you can choose to move forward into a more joyous moment and an even more positive future. You can take a step at a time and begin forgiving those who have transgressed you and judged you. Feel how you feel when you have forgiven those who have transgressed and judged you."

Destiny follows Alice's forgiveness process and then speaks excitedly to Alice,

"I found an early event where I started to rely on others feedback to formulate who I should be. When I observed my memory of that early event, I realised that it happened differently than I remembered. I was able to make the event mean something different. Then I forgave someone who had a significant impact in that event, and then I forgave myself for listening to others feedback about who they think I am because I now know that what I think of me is what matters. I feel like I have taken that first step to change my focus on what I think of myself. I have changed my memory through changing my belief because I have changed my thinking around what I thought the past should have been. I have changed my emotions that link to my memories so that those old emotions will not leak into my future. I have chosen to leave the old emotions in the past where they belong. I can feel that change has happened within me after the forgiveness process. I have released the negatives in my life, which changed how I was thinking around that situation that ultimately changed my experiences. For example, their malicious gossip became their malicious gossip, not mine. I have now freed myself to imagine a happier future. I don't have that heavy feeling of resentment. My heavy emotions have lifted, and I feel like I have taken a step away from the event to be the observer without emotion. It's gone."

Happy tears were streaming down Destiny's cheeks. Destiny sat for a moment and then took three deep breaths and sat quietly to listen to Alice.

Opportunities and possibilities - the second step

"Opportunities and possibilities are the second steps towards reaching your end goal. You can choose from your many choices to change your focus from what you hear and how others colour your world. You can choose to change your focus to rely on listening to your feedback to appreciate you to colour your own world. You can choose from your choices to be the designer of your life to become the best version of yourself. Would you like to do that?" asks Alice.

Destiny thinks for a moment and then says,

"Yes, that would be awesome."

Alice begins her spiel,

"When you become aware of the many possibilities and opportunities available to you to choose your change, what will you choose?"

Destiny takes her time to explore her thoughts.

"I sense that I don't have to remain the same because I can change my focus to believe that I can discover the many opportunities and possibilities available to me now. When I change my belief to what I can do, I change my focus to be aware of the many possibilities and opportunities that have always been there for me. I can make a list and prioritise who I need to be to do the job that I desire, including the steps I need to take to attract a connected staff and variety in my work. I can work towards attracting a job that values me," says Destiny excitedly.

"Excellent," says Alice.

Courage - the third step

"Courage is the third step towards changing your focus. Use courage to go with the ebb and flow of the experience of life and follow your heart to make your dreams come true. The flow of life may give you twists and turns and even block your way. With courage, you can choose, and you will have the awareness to know which way to follow and which way not to follow and how to change what isn't working to enjoy your journey as you progress towards your destination. You can have the courage to receive feedback and do something different to act on that feedback," says Alice.

"I can re-discover my inner courage to be aware and curious around my choices that will grow my self-confidence and build my self-esteem. I will cope more effectively with a narcissist whilst following my heart and intellect to find suitable job prospects for me. I can distract my focus from the narcissist and focus on me. I could even work on immediate change and add more exercise and meditation to my daily habits to distract me from focusing on others behaviour. I can influence myself and not focus on others influencing me. I can confidently choose to know what works for me, what doesn't work for me and what I need or can choose to change," says Destiny.

"What else would you need for your desired change?" asks Alice.

Destiny thinks for a moment. She stares at the wall in front of her, on that spot just above her direct vision. She draws in a deep breath and exhales excitedly,

Understanding - the fourth step

"When I understand that I have the power and flexibility to change my choice for my change repeatedly until I have the change that serves me, and then I can choose to change it again. I can choose my choice for my change anytime that I want to. When I change my thoughts to change my feelings and emotions, I directly affect my behaviour and thoughts, which means that I can be the designer of my life because I will know what I can influence and what I won't let influence me," says Destiny.

"Well done, you've got this." congratulates Alice,

"What else will you do to change your focus to have what you need to be the version you choose to be to have the life of your choice?" asks Alice.

Self-talk and self-love. Being who you choose to be - the fifth step.

"When I harness my heart, my body and my brain's power, I can achieve my choice for change because it is not just what we do for a change. It is how we are different that makes the difference," says Destiny.

"Awesome work, Destiny," says Alice.

"What else do you need to do to have the change that will create the best version of you?" asks Alice.

Destiny thinks for a moment and then responds,

"I can practice gratitude. I can spend time every morning writing a list of what I am grateful for and include my gratitudes in my journaling every evening. I can commit to doing this for a month as a start."

"That's excellent, Destiny," Congratulates Alice,

"I remember reading that the law of attraction says that what you focus on is what you get. Gratitude begets gratitude. Destiny, you can use the FOCUS program to change at a deeper level where you break through your negative emotions and limiting beliefs to change them so you don't bleed them into now and your future. You can change your direction to be who you need to be to heal yourself, recover and create the best version of yourself. I want to share with you a quote that may resonate with you.

Gratitude unlocks the fullness of life. It turns what we have into enough and more. It turns denial into acceptance, chaos to order, confusion to clarity.-Melody Beattie (https://melodybeattie.com/gratitude-2/)

Change your focus to feel the fear and release it whilst being grateful for everything that surrounds you. Fears are the gatekeepers to our greatest gifts. Fear is a warning that there is change approaching and alerts you to move ahead with care. If it is a warning of something dangerous, then take care. If not, then find your courage to move forward and find your internal warrior," says Alice,

"Now, tell me what you have learned so far."

Destiny twists her hair between her forefinger and her thumb, creases her brow and then says,

"I have learned that forgiveness is vital for me because it is through forgiveness that I can change my feelings to set me free to make informed decisions for me to choose the choice for my change. I can release the feelings of hurt to free me up to get back to that place of love within me. I can forgive myself for letting storytellers design my life instead of taking responsibility to be the architect of my life."

"Well done," says Alice, "Can I share with you that forgiveness is for self and not for the person that holds the resentment. They don't even have to know that you have forgiven them. You can forgive yourself too for relying on others feedback to mould you as a person and create your life in the workplace. Forgive yourself and forgive others. Then forgiveness is freeing.

We are born to access specific resources that we need to function in life, so choose carefully. Our feelings and emotions are gifts that can guide us to perceive then to conceive something new. We can choose our feelings and emotions that give us the ability to love, heal, and imagine. Our emotions can create our life. We can choose from all of our feelings, knowing that every one of them is here to serve us. What else can you tell me?" Alice asks Destiny.

Destiny thinks for a moment and then says,

"Forgiveness is about me feeling my emotions and choosing which ones to acknowledge, release and clear. It is more than an idea or an intention to say I forgive that person. Forgiveness needs to happen at a deeper level to choose to change my emotions at a deeper level. I can then free myself from the unchanged emotions and bring my chosen emotions into the now and the future."

Alice commends Destiny and says,

"Excellent. Yes, that's right. Our culture tells us to get over it and move on. It doesn't work that way because we are more emotional than people think we are. Go slowly to feel your feelings of hurt, sadness, anger and other feelings without hurting yourself or others. Go through a process and let it out of your body, and that's when we can truly forgive. Learn to connect with your pain, and then let it go. If we don't, we suppress the heaviness and push away our light where our creativity lives.

Forgiving is a way to get back to that place of love within us.

We're not supposed to hang on to our emotions. **How do we let go of our emotions?** We observe them, feel them, feel them in our bodies, and then feel the change in our bodies as those emotions release from our bodies.

What else did you discover?" asks Alice.

Destiny responds,

"I get it. If I do not change my negative emotions and do that through the forgiveness process, I will suppress them. When I store my emotions, I hold both negative with positive emotions, and I suppress them down into layers. If I remain the same, I will attract the same and miss the many opportunities and possibilities available to me.

I can change my focus to choose the thoughts that will allow me to maintain an optimistic attitude and free me to be positive. If I focus on forgiveness to change my feelings, I will set my soul free. I can focus on gratitude to change my feelings that change my emotions that can heal my past and influence who I want to be today."

Alice interrupts the silence and says,

"You can shift your focus through forgiveness and practising gratitude towards remaining optimistically positive. Giving you clarity around who you want to be, to take the action that aligns with your values, provides you with the power to design your way forward to go with the flow of life towards your chosen outcome. Choose how you would like to ride your boat in your river of life. Focus on your now and your future."

"I choose to have gratitude for now and a healthy outlook for what I imagine for the future that can be", responds Destiny.

"Would you like me to take you through a forgiveness relaxation hypnosis where you use self-hypnosis?" asks Alice.

Destiny nods.

Forgiveness

"Find a place to sit quietly and comfortably to enhance your physical and mental relaxation.

Close your eyes and let your body relax.

Notice how you can feel your breath, and you are breathing in deeply and breathing out any tension to enhance your physical relaxation.

Breathe softly and naturally.

You can feel your feet relax and feel the relaxation creep into your toes.

You sense your legs relaxing, relaxing your calves and relaxing your thighs more and more.

See how relaxed you feel and experience the tingly warm feeling of relaxation in your legs travelling up your body into your pelvis.

Relax your abdomen, and then relax your stomach muscles.

Feel that relaxed tingly feeling and watch it travel up your spine, relaxing each and every vertebra.

You are deeply relaxed. Deeper and deeper and deeper than before.

Feel your heartbeat and sense your heart space opening like a rosebud opens into a beautifully perfumed rose.

Relax your lungs and sense the tingly warm feeling relaxing your shoulders and travelling down your arms into everyone one of your fingers and down into your fingertips.

Relax your neck and feel your face relax your forehead and your whole body is relaxed.

Feel your eyelids close gently.

Relax and go deeper.

Breathe in deeply and out. Feel your mind relax.

You hear yourself say, relax, mental mind. It is your turn to relax and continue breathing softly and naturally.

You imagine your favourite comfortable, relaxing place, go there now.

On the count of three, you will be in your favourite place where you notice what is in front of you, what is beside you, what is behind you in this peaceful, relaxing, comfortable space.

Is there motion in the air, or is the air still.

Are there any sounds in your place of relaxation, or is this a place of silence?

Can you smell the flavours floating in the air for you to taste?

Imagine you have more and more time in the world to spend here. Relax deeper.

Breathe in deeply and out, and know that you are relaxed and ready to program your mind even deeper.

You are now at the starting point to use your mind to choose your choices and make changes.

See a staircase in front of you with ten steps.

Stand on the top of the stairs and count back from 10 to 1 as you take each step. 10, 9 going deeper and deeper within, 8,7 deeper and deeper feel yourself going deeper and deeper 6,5,4,3, deeper and deeper and more deeper 2, deeper and deeper. Relax more and more. Relax even deeper, deeper and deeper. 1. You are there.

Take a slow healthy deep breath and as you exhale, feel how relaxed you are now.

You are always in control and can accept or choose any level of the mind.

You are in control. If anyone calls you, you will be awake and in the room to answer.

Take a deep breath, and as you exhale and relax even more.

Find yourself standing in a particular place where the blue azure sea meets the white silicon sand.

Hear the clear azure blue water gently lapping the white silicon sand.

Feel the sand moving under your feet, and feel the grains of sand between your toes.

In the distance, you see your guide building a cleansing fire.

You can see the flames dancing to the tune of a love song holding each other close.

The white and red flames are licking the sides of the safe purpose-built black steel fire pit, reaching out with love to take your release of tension, negative thoughts, negative feelings and negative emotions.

Imagine that you are sitting with your guide on the pure white silicon sand by the fire pit. Way over there on the other side of the fire pit, you look over the firepit at the sand, and you sense the historical event with the attached emotions you choose to release.

You see that past you, the younger you sitting with the person who caused the emotions, you need to forgive. You can hear them talking about the emotions filled with sadness, anger, guilt and frustration.

Imagine that you are watching from way back here whilst the younger you faces the other person sitting beside her way over there.

Listen as the younger you says what she needs to say to the other person.

Let the younger you talk until there is nothing left to say, then let the other person say what he/she needs to say until there is nothing more to say.

Ask the younger you if she is ready to forgive.

If yes, let her say I may not condone what you did. I forgive you from the bottom of my heart. I know that you can learn to understand what you did and forgive yourself, then watch the younger you as she watches the other person disappear into the cleansing fire, releasing the tension, negative thoughts, feelings and emotions.

When you are ready, ask the younger you to share her learnings and bring them back into the now.

Take note of the learnings.

Now you can turn to the younger you and let her know that she now has the learnings and resources to understand and resourcefully cope with the event. Now you can let the younger you grow back into you with her selected resources installed.

You can open your arms and welcome her back into you.

Ask the guide if there is anything more to add. Sometimes it will be advice or a simple nod.

If the younger you cannot forgive, that's okay.

The younger you can say something like, I don't condone your behaviour, and I hope you learn what you have done and learn to forgive yourself.

When you sense that the younger you has said all that she needs to say, let her take her learnings. And as you sit by the fire, you watch the younger you sit peacefully and watch the other person walk into the cleansing fire of love, confidentiality and forgiveness.

You may need to forgive your younger you and let her know that she can forgive when she is ready.

Embrace your younger you.

You can choose to forgive your younger you. And let your younger you know that you didn't have the resources then that you have now. Let the older you say what she needs to say and then invite the younger you to grow into the older you. You may want to hug the younger you.

Imagine seeing you and your guide, putting out the fire and walking back along the beach.

You can feel the smooth silicon sand granules under your feet and in between your toes.

You walk towards the water that beckons you. You place one toe into the water and then your foot.

You can feel the purity of silicon cleansed water flowing over your feet as they sink into the wet silicon particles of sand below.

You can feel the water cleansing all of you as you walk out deeper and deeper.

You sense that safe feeling when the silky softness of the water envelopes you.

You are lighter, even more, lighter than before. So light you feel yourself floating on the clear blue azure sea's surface. You hear the lapping of the water around and taste the salty cleansing taste of the water that flows so softly.

You feel appreciation and gratitude radiating from every cell in your body.

When you think of that event now, you can see it without feeling the pain?

You walk towards the stairs, and when you reach the bottom, you turn to your guide and thank him for helping you release the pain.

Take the first step, then the second, the third, the fourth, the fifth, the sixth, the seventh.

Slowly and gently bring yourself back to this time and know that you may not know that you have all the resources you need, and these resources are installed within you now.

Step on the eighth step, nine and ten.

Now you are back in the room. Open your eyes when you are ready. Feel how peaceful and relaxed that you feel.

How do you feel now?" asks Alice.

"I feel light, empowered and confident to cope with events as they present."

"How do you feel about that old situation now?" asks Alice

"I feel unattached. I can't find that old emotion to feel it."

"Excellent. Can you imagine a time in the next month when you might be in a similar work situation? What happens, and how do you react?" asks Alice

"I can see that same situation, and I tell myself that it's not my issue to own," says Destiny.

"Excellent. Can you imagine a time in the next three months when you might be in a similar work situation? What happens, and how do you react?" asks Alice

"I can see that same situation, and I sense that it's not my issue to own," says Destiny.

"Excellent. Can you imagine a time in the next six months when you might be in a similar situation? What happens, and how do you react?" asks Alice

"I can see that same work situation, and I know it's not my issue to own," says Destiny.

"Well done. Are you ready right now to be the architect of the rest of your life? You can choose right now, from the many opportunities available to you to have a design of your choice?" says Alice

Opportunities

"That would be excellent. I could draw my future by designing a **vision board** to help me see where I want to be. I can add a written list of specific elements that I need to contribute to my end design. My friend, Tania, designed her vision board using images of the partner she wished to attract. She had it hanging in a prominent place in her home, a place where she could sit and see it every day. Tania said that she valued the guidance her vision board gave her. And as she designed her vision board that kept her on track with creating her future, she used her awareness to reflect on her past to use her learnings to enrich her life's design. Tania became aware of her happiness emotions right now and decided to take them into her future. She imagined what makes her happy and included those images in her vision board.

Tania also wrote down a specific and detailed description of him. She folded the paper which she left in her bedside drawer. Every day Tania looked at her vision board and imagined feeling her emotions of achieving her dreams. Tania imagined, feeling the powerful energy that created her thoughts that made her emotions that she would feel when she was with the partner of her dreams. Tania sensed what it felt like to have her dream partner with her already. Tania listened to the exciting conversations around her, and she could hear her self talk. She could taste the food she was sharing with good company and smell the inviting aroma wafting around her. Tania met someone who met 90% of the elements in her design. He measured up, and they had a long and happy relationship. They pooled their money to buy a house of their creation. They found a place that matched most of their vision board pictures and met even more of their written criteria. They went ahead with the purchase and made it their home. I can do this for work because I now know that there are many jobs available for me." says Destiny.

Alice listens and observes the excitement radiating from Destiny. Alice then says,

"If you create a vision board to align your ideas with your thoughts to design your feelings and emotions, then you can make the plan for the ideal life for you that will encourage your unconscious mind to support you to live your design for your life. When looking at your vision board, use all of your senses to bring your vision to life as if it is real right now. Balance your life and change your focus to change your thoughts to create the life of your dreams. Be courageous and know that it's okay to feel your emotions and choose which emotions to keep and which feelings to release to have a balanced life of your design."

Destiny listens intently and then says,

"I can create a vision board that represents all of my achievements to remind me of my capability and inspire me to move to a place where I can do that again. I could include pictures, poems and inspirational quotes to generate my feelings of knowing that I am enough as I am right now. That's right, and I can.

I believe that great strength lies within love, and just as much great power lies within anger and hate. When feelings of despair surround me, I think that the solution would be to draw these feelings even closer, to embrace them, draw them into me, feel them cleanly, and then they will naturally release.

I can choose to feel my emotions to free them continually. If I keep my feelings clean without the story, then I will have my life's power. I can choose to ignore my social conditioning of being told, "Don't feel your emotions." I can feel all of them cleanly and keep and release as I choose. I can be the architect of my thoughts to determine my feelings and emotions to match my desired responses to challenging situations.

My emotions are the lens through which I sense my world. Feelings are my life's power source. I can create power just by feeling my feelings, and I need emotions to live because they motivate me. They provide a necessary pathway for my personal growth. The more I value my feelings, the more I love myself, and the more I love myself, the more I appreciate my feelings, and there is so much emotional energy that lives and flows within me.

All of the painful personal feelings that I experience come from not allowing the flow of emotions. Once my feelings flow into me, I know that I have to feel them. I can choose to observe my feelings and emotions passing through me or choose to keep them. I am the architect of my life. I can be the best version of me."

"Well done for expanding your awareness to see the many possibilities and opportunities that are available to you," says Alice.

Destiny responds excitedly, "I can focus on the many opportunities that are available to me and know what they mean to guide me forward. I can design my goals to give me meaning in my life and take the steps, even baby steps towards achieving my goals."

Courage

The next time Destiny meets with Alice, and Destiny tells Alice,

"I sense the many more opportunities that are available to me right now, and I believe that I have found my courage to keep choosing until I find the opportunities and possibilities that work for me. I have the confidence and feel that my self-esteem is growing to support me in my adventures to find the change that is most suited to me."

Destiny's eyes sparkle with nervous excitement as she commits to moving towards her significant outcome of finding her happiness,

"I won't let anyone stand in my way. I will please me and keep myself safe. I have the courage. I know how to find my limiting beliefs, and I know how to change them. If I change my perception of an event in the past, I can change my thoughts to change my feelings and emotions. I can choose to be strong and back myself to succeed,"

Destiny stops to draw breath. She pushes her hair back from her forehead and says,

"I am so grateful to find that I do have the courage to shift my focus through forgiveness and practising gratitude. I can change my thoughts to change my feelings and emotions to give me a choice to maintain a positive attitude for my journey. I have the courage to see what works; eliminate what doesn't work; know that I can create something different as many times as I need to until my life choices align with my values and purpose. I know I am repeating myself because I am excited to feel empowered and have a deep understanding of this. I can influence the change in how I see my environment around me." Destiny takes a deep breath and smiles radiantly. Destiny turns to Alice and says,

"Thank you for your guidance to find my courage, to embrace my opportunities and feel the release of emotions through the forgiveness process."

Alice congratulates Destiny for finding her courage to propel herself forward and choose to design a life of excellence.

Understanding

"I understand that I can make changes at an unconscious level to change at a conscious level to change my life even more efficiently. I can do this through self-hypnosis as I did for the forgiveness process. I understand that I can change my fears to gratitude and appreciation to release the endorphins that make me feel happy and better every day. I think that feeling better and better every day is a bonus. Through self-hypnosis, I can now make changes at an unconscious level to change at a conscious level to change my thoughts that change my feelings even more easily. I understand that I can even change my limiting beliefs and embedded beliefs. If I change my thoughts that change my feelings, I can control what happens internally and choose to go with my external environment's flow. I can flow with outside influences and know that I can influence how I respond. I can choose to influence myself to choose to maintain a positive attitude."

Destiny stops to think about a time in her past when she had influenced her inner thoughts to maintain a positive attitude to survive a significant health issue.

"I can model me," said Destiny. She breaths, she laughs and then she smiles.

Alice gives Destiny space to experience her aha moments and celebrate them then Alice says,

"Just know that painful emotions like fear can be a warning that change is happening. It means that you need to move away from the snake that you see sunning itself on the path you are walking, or it can mean that change is happening, so take care and be aware as you move forward. Sometimes emotions are signs to provide feedback when your life is out of balance.

Your feelings can let you know when something is wrong and something needs to change. You can use fear to serve you. You can decide to change fearful, nervous feelings into nervous excitement. Emotions bring us pleasure and pain, and we can choose for ourselves what we want to feel. You can't turn off your feelings, but you can select your feelings. You can choose to use your feelings for good and not manipulate your feelings into twisted and false emotions through the story. You made me sad can be changed to I feel sad, and that is where our power lies. When our thinking creates our feelings, we can change our feelings when we change our thinking. Easy really. It's just the habit that pulls us back.

Understand that with self-hypnosis guidance, you can make changes effortlessly at an unconscious level to change at a conscious level to change your thoughts that change your feelings to maintain a positive attitude even more now. You know that you may find this a hard habit to break if you suppress your emotions or manipulate your feelings. When you are ready, you can create an energetic behavioural change to change a habit through self-hypnosis that makes the change even more rapidly."

Destiny thinks for a moment and says,

"I've seen hypnosis on television. I laughed at some of the antics. Does that mean it only works on unsuspecting people?"

"No hypnosis is **self-hypnosis** that is a state that we experience every day. Self- hypnosis is a natural state that we experience every day when we wake in the morning and just before we fall asleep at night. We're in a self-hypnosis state during the day at times, like when you drive to work every day and wonder if you stopped at the red light or was it green. When you think about it, you remember that you don't even remember the trip from home to work. Watching television puts us into a hypnotic state, where we internalise information received, so we need to be careful with what we watch.

Daydreaming is a self-hypnotic state where you are miles away, and when you hear your name, you are brought back in that room. The self-hypnosis state happens when your brain waves slow from the beta level (our conscious level) to the alpha level (unconscious level), where we can make changes quickly. We can make quick and effective habit changes, change our negative emotions and discover a state where we can change our limiting beliefs," says Alice

"You mean that the self-hypnotic state is powerful, and I can be my powerhouse because I am in control of me and my mind the whole time?" asks Destiny.

Alice responds,

"Yes. No one can control your mind. It is not mind control. The CIA experimented unsuccessfully with mind control in their MKUltra project in the 1950s. https://en.wikipedia. org/wiki/Project_MKUltra.

Hypnosis is safe, and it is a skill that everyone should learn. You will feel relaxed, so relaxed that you can effectively engage your imagination to visualise and make change even more quickly at an unconscious level. It's important to remember that you are in control during the hypnosis process. You are 100% responsible for your hypnosis experience. You are responsible for relaxing your body, and all you have to do is follow instruction, and you can can't you follow instruction.

Your unconscious mind has many prime directives. It stores and organises memories, represses memories with unresolved negative emotions, presents repressed memories for resolution and may keep suppressed emotions hidden for protection. Your unconscious mind runs the body, preserves the body, is the domain of your feelings, enjoys serving, and needs clear orders to follow and even more.

We all form beliefs in our early years in our unconscious mind that we bring with us on our life's journey. Some of those beliefs serve us, and others can hold us back. We can choose to be selective to change the ones we wish to change and keep those we believe will serve us now and into our future. We can make this change even more quickly using hypnosis, where we slow our brain waves into the Alpha level just like we do right before sleep and when we wake first thing in the morning. That is in our unconscious mind, where we form our habits and create change even more quickly for the conscious mind to engage."

Destiny closes her eyes. She wriggles in her seat to make herself more comfortable when she says,

"So if I want, I can change my belief around being a people pleaser. Sometimes, I feel like I am pushing the proverbial uphill in my workplace because sometimes, no matter what I do, I can't do what other people expect of me? I feel that I'm not good enough to be liked, and then I think I am failing at my job. You mean, I can change my feelings of self-doubt and change my emotions even more quickly using self - hypnosis?"

Alice smiles and says,

"Yes, you can. If you feel negative emotions around your co-workers or your boss, you can think of the thoughts that come up like I am not good enough to be liked, or you may feel self-doubt feelings arising from your thoughts. Raise your awareness to think about the feelings that arise for you and identify your thoughts that bring up those feelings. You can repeat this process, or you can journal. Write whatever comes into your head and then review to look for patterns of feelings and emotions. Acknowledge them, feel them intensely, and release those that you choose to remove. Emotions will pass through you unless you decide to keep them."

Destiny's eyes widen, and she responds excitedly,

"If I think that I am excluded and feel sad, then I can focus on the feeling of sadness and then it will pass?" asks Destiny

"Yes, and as you focus on the emotion, let any thoughts of story pass you by, and the emotion will pass too then you can choose the thoughts that will give you the emotion of your choosing," says Alice.

"Wow, I feel so much lighter knowing that I have a lot more control than I thought," exclaims Destiny.

"Excellent," responds Alice and then is quick to continue,

"If you focus on your self-talk to be kind to yourself, to build your certainty in self-belief, to synchronise your life with your values, then you can master your mind and change your feelings. You can be who you choose to be, do what you can do, and have the feelings you choose to have an optimistic mindset to maintain a positive attitude moving forward.

Did you know that everyone talks to themselves? You are the one who spends the most time with you, and you are the one who talks to you the most. When you think of self-talk, it's like thinking about your thoughts. You can change your thoughts, and you can change your self-talk. What if you could manage your negative self-talk and then choose to have positive self-talk instead?" asks Alice.

Destiny allows herself time to think about Alice's musings and says,

"I remember a time when I was eight years old, and I was enjoying the fun at the local swimming pool. I can see myself standing on the edge of the three-metre board, ready to dive into the water below. I remember the excitement and confidence I felt when taking up the challenge to climb the ladder. And then I remember how my emotions changed to fear when I arrived at the top of the three-metre-board and saw what was beneath me. I can still sense that feeling of self – doubt and fear that crept into me. I remember that I began to argue with myself. Yes, I can do it. No, you can't. You haven't dived from this height before. What if you do a belly flop that will hurt? I can dive. I know I can. I dive in from the side of the pool every time I come for a swim. This board is just a bit higher. No, you can't. You will hurt yourself. I don't want to hurt myself. I am up here now, and I'm not climbing back down that ladder."

I remember that I changed my fear to meet the challenge. I changed my focus to notice that I was taking a deep breath. I extended my arms high above my head and jumped high. I can remember feeling the strength I felt when I leapt and dived an almost perfect dive. I remember feeling exhilarated, and then I climbed back up the ladder to do it again. If I had listened to my discouraging negative self-talk, I would not have dived, and I would have missed an exhilarating experience that I enjoyed so much that I repeated that dive over and over again. I would have missed my experience of courage that inspired me to repeat it over and over again," Destiny excitedly tells Alice.

Alice observes Destiny's expression change from a wrinkled brow of concern to a smile etching its way across her face. Then Alice says,

"You may think that you are crazy for having negative self-talk. I believe that it was trying to keep you the same to keep you safe from the threat out there. Maybe that space of judgment between the conscious and unconscious mind filling your negative self-talk wanted to stop you from feeling embarrassed. Psychology recognises it as a thing and calls it negative bias, which means that we are inclined to see what is wrong more than what is right is."

Alice pauses to give Destiny time to absorb this information, then she continues,

"Firstly, you need to be aware of your self-talk and accept that it is the way it is. Secondly, you need to make space to fill with positive self-talk, and you can do this through gratitude as it is one of the subsets of love, and we all strive for love in our lives. Did you know that you can't have love and fear at the same time? So choose love and instil positive self-talk and don't give any energy to negative talk. Reduce your negative chatter and then remove it. Let yourself off the hook and know that you can manage your negative self-talk and replace it with peace and with space. If you decide to, you can do this by encouraging positivity and validating. Say thank you, but I understand negativity is not for me at the moment because I have decided to choose the positivity of love. I acknowledge that I am enough and that I am where I am supposed to be. I know that I can change negative self-talk to have positive self – talk. I understand that I am not my self-talk. I have self-talk, which means I have an awareness of self-talk. We get to choose the relationship that we have our self-talk."

Destiny listens and thinks for a moment before responding,

"If I accept my self-talk, I can let my negative thoughts pass and make space to choose gratitude to create as much love space as I can. I can do this when my negative thoughts come up. When I think that I am not good enough, I can accept that thought and then I can choose to take my power to say thank you, but I choose to know that I am enough. When negative thoughts come up, I will say that I choose not to give energy to my negative thoughts through the narrative of self-talk, and it will weaken my negative self-talk. It will eventually go away, and I can create space for positivity. Of course, I will not argue with my self-talk as I did on the diving board because that is a waste of energy. I know that when a negative thought comes up that I now know that I am not my negative thought, and that is where my power lies, and I know that I can do this anywhere in any situation."

"Excellent work, Destiny," says Alice,

"You can be kind to yourself through self-talk, and you can build your certainty in self-belief and self-love so that you can master your mind. When you master your mind, amazing things happen. Kindness and loving self -talk changes how you feel and how you feel changes your chemical reaction. Be kind to yourself through self-talk and build your certainty in self-belief to master your mind and change your feelings to be who you choose to be and do what you can do to have the sense you choose.

Shine through gratitude and appreciation and raise your endorphins, those happy chemicals that you have within you now. We are, after all, electrical impulses that create chemical reactions. Create those chemicals within you now that makes you feel better and better every day in every way.

Lead yourself, to learn to grow and to love to have the freedom to choose your choice for your change.

Appreciate what you have now, and believe in yourself," suggests Alice.

Belief in self

Destiny spent time processing Alice's information sharing. At the next meeting, Destiny shares her insights,

"I have changed my beliefs to flavour my self-talk. I choose to believe that:

I am the power in my world,

I flow with the change taking place in my life as best I can,

I approve of myself and the way I am changing,

I am doing the best I can,

I am worthy of the very best life, and now I lovingly allow myself to accept it,

I love and approve of myself,

I trust the process of life,

I relax into the flow of energy,

I go beyond the limitations of my memes and my mind viruses,

I am free to be the best I can,

I align my choices with my values. I draw on all the resources that I have within me to grow, earn, learn, and love.

And I love the words of Viktor Frankl:

When we no longer can change a situation, then we need to change ourselves (Viktor Frankl)
https://www.dailygood.org/story/1578/

I believe that I can work on changing myself. If I spend time and spend an hour of power each day that I dedicate to self-development, then I will be able to choose my way forward on my terms."

Destiny remembers reading a University of Woollongong article about workplace bullying and then says,

"I have control of how I think and what I feel. I can't control what is happening in my external environment. I know that research is happening around workplace bullying because it is a significant issue in many countries, including Australia. Recently available research indicates that nearly half of all Australian employees have experienced workplace bullying at some stage during their working life. Workplace bullying has implications for the mental and physical health and well-being of employees and organisations. Bullied staff can experience depression, anxiety, and physical health conditions such as hypertension. I know that bullying can affect teamwork because I have seen motivation drop. I've watched people take massive amounts of sick leave or leave searching for a better job. And I wonder why I see the bully stay and the bullied almost always leave?"

Destiny fiddles with her hair twirling it between her thumb and forefinger, then she continues,

"I can choose to stay, or I can choose to run. I can choose my change, and I can permit myself to be my hero in my story. I can decide to shift my focus to change my thoughts' meaning to select my choice of feelings. If I stop, take a deep breath and then respond instead of reacting instantly, I can choose my ideas to create my choice's emotions. I really can choose to stay or leave," espouses Destiny

"Excellent work, Destiny," commends Alice,

"You are the architect of your life, and you can begin by identifying your desired outcome and designing the steps to take towards reaching your chosen end goal.

Know your OUTCOME. What do you want?

Align with your values. Identify what is most important to you and then identify the next important step and what is next and then the next and align your outcome to your values. If integrity is essential, then align with people and organisations that value integrity. You can choose your choice for your change and know that you can back yourself to achieve your desired outcome. You can choose to stay and be your authentic self where you choose your feelings to serve you, or you can choose your choice from all of the opportunities and possibilities that are out there for your change."

Love what you are doing today or change it. Shift your FOCUS to change your thoughts to honour yourself. You can break through your stuckness of embedded beliefs and negative decisions to feel empowered to move forward. And as you move through your discomfort to break through the barriers of growth, you will know that you will find your true transformation through awareness. The mammalian part of your brain will try to pull you back to keep you the same to keep you safe, and you will know to tell your mammalian brain that you can make your own decisions to change your focus to back yourself whilst you keep moving forward. You can choose from the opportunities available to you out there to leave, or you can develop your resilience even more, to choose to stay and confidently move forward.

Life is like a bicycle. To keep your balance, keep moving –Albert Einstein. (https://quoteinvestigator.com/2015/06/28/bicycle/)

CHAPTER SIX

Turquoise – Men at work misbehaving; from hurt to healing

"Yes, it seems to be me that they are good at getting rid of old ladies past their use-by date. And as I go into battle, I must keep my self-esteem intact and build my confidence to survive," says Turquoise quietly to herself as she walks towards her mentor's workspace.

"Hello, Turquoise, how are you today?" asks Connie, who is Turquoise's coach and mentor.

"I'm okay, thank you, Connie," responds Turquoise and then shifts to make herself comfortable in her seat in the middle of the oversized couch that she has to herself. She takes time to look around Connie's room and sees Connie facing her. Connie sits on her chair with her back to her desk where her computer sits. Connie notices the scenic prints on the walls and the soft light filtering through the soft window curtaining. The door is closed shut, and the environment feels comfortable and inviting, with a salt light shining softly on the table in the corner. Turquoise can smell the sweet scent of red roses that reminds her of her childhood freedoms. Connie is an older lady with neatly cut, greying hair. She wears designer glasses that match her multi-coloured hippie outfit. Connie exudes warmth and smiles comfortingly, then asks,

"What can we help you with today, Turquoise?" asks Connie.

"I feel like I need to go into battle with the boys who are getting rid of old ladies past their use-by date. I need to overcome my fear and self-doubt to preserve my self-confidence and relieve my lower back pain," says Turquoise.

"Do you have back pain right now?" asks Connie.

"Yes, I do. I try to ignore it, but sometimes the pain overwhelms me," says Turquoise.

"Just wondered if you would like to try a quick process to help with your back pain?" asks Connie.

Turquoise nods.

"Ask yourself what emotion am I feeling now?" asks Connie.

Turquoise wriggles in her seat, wrinkles her brow and scrunches her face, and then she closes her eyes and sits quietly as if she is processing her feelings. Time passes, and then Turquoise opens her eyes and smiles.

"How do you feel now?" asks Connie.

"I feel a bit more relaxed, and the pain has eased. Wow. I feel calm, and I feel better," says Turquoise.

"That's right. Can you tell me more about the boys and why you need to go into battle with them," asks Connie.

"I have fallen into the pattern of trusting and showing my vulnerability through misplaced friendship just like I did with Golly. Well, at a different level. I suspect that Beastie, my friend, is now my enemy because he supports Grim, who supports Slippery Jim, who supports Big Red to get rid of old ladies past their use-by date.

I'm approaching my mid-forties, so I guess that is me,"

Turquoise sighs loudly and then continues,

"I know that I'm old enough to say no and mean it. That is when I feel strong. It feels like another part of me lets self-doubt creep in, and I notice that my strong feeling leaves me."

Turquoise stares at the opposite wall whilst she twirls her long strands of hair between her forefinger and thumb and then says,

"Did I tell you that Beastie said that he knows that I can get through this because of what I have already survived?"

Turquoise stops to take a breath, and then she continues,

"He asks me if I go home and kick the dog because of what we are doing to you."

Connie nods and listens while intently focusing on Turquoise. She gives Turquoise space to think, and then Turquoise resumes her speak,

"I have learned to react differently and take a deep breath and say nothing to Beastie and tell myself that he projects his emotional issues by trying to make them mine, and then I take another deep breath and choose to feel my choice of feeling, just like you showed me. Sometimes I will quietly say that I don't kick the dog because I love my dog, and that is when Beastie grimaces and walks away, and I have to say that at the point, I feel empowered."

Connie waits for Turquoise to finish speaking and then says,

"You can't change other people's feelings, and you can't stop them from intentionally trying to influence your emotional state. You can deflect their attempts to influence you. You can instead choose to listen to you, and your thoughts that choose your emotions, so well done," congratulates Connie.

Turquoise has lots more to say,

"I did feel challenged when Grim told me that Slippery Jim referred to getting rid of older ladies past their use-by date. I made that mean that there would be a focus on restructuring my area. When I took the time to remember, I realised that I had noticed how many older ladies had left work, sold up, and moved away. At the time, it didn't occur to me that they may be targeting me too."

Connie gives Turquoise space to think. When Turquoise is ready, she continues,

"I initially felt confused when there was a push to ignore any references to my achievements, but I didn't think that my job would become redundant or that the executive of this newly formed regime would view me as redundant. I thought my achievements would value add to this newly formed institution, but they just didn't want to know. I felt burned, and I felt like they were dragging me back into the middle of the last century, and I wasn't going quietly. You know, sometimes Beastie surprises me with directives to achieve highly. I'm not fussed about surprises, and when I least expect, he expects me to perform at a level that he refused to work. Beastie ignored my comment that he had refused to do the same. He just shook his head, pointed his finger and told me that I just had to do it. When I think about it, Beastie knows me well enough to know my buttons to press, and Beastie consistently pushes hard to push me over the edge and out. I can feel the push because my back hurt, and my self –esteem has dropped. My body is trying to tell me that it is having a chemical reaction to my emotions too. Even so, I don't want to leave on his terms. I am determined to leave on my terms. I do have commitments, just like everyone else."

Turquoise takes a few deep breaths to ground herself. Then Connie says,

"I believe that if you want to stay, you will need to build your resilience even more strongly for the time you have left working here."

"How do I do that?" asks Turquoise.

"If it is okay with you, can I share with you what I think may help you?" Connie asks Turquoise.

Turquoise nods in agreement. Connie says,

"What if you were to set boundaries around what you will tolerate and accept. Remember that if the men at work misbehaving won't respect your feelings, needs and boundaries, you can. You can decide not to take on their words when they use their words to unsettle you. Maybe it would help to know that if you are easily insulted, then you are easily manipulated. I suggest that you remember to take a deep breath before responding to align with your boundaries that you can frame with your purpose and values?"

Connie pauses to give Turquoise space. Connie then says,

"And as you elicit your values and set your goals to create meaning in your life, you can design a roadmap towards your desired destination. You can include the detours along the way. The first is setting boundaries for what you will accept and what you won't accept from the 'Men at work misbehaving'. Each time you accomplish a goal or successfully negotiate a detour, you can make it mean that you are one step closer to where you want to be."

Turquoise is quick to respond,

"Okay, I will date my goal for six months. If today is the 20th of June and now 2.30 pm, I set my goal for 20th December at 2.30 pm when I open my paysheet and see that my pay has increased by 40% and I deposit $500 into my bank account. On the 20th of December at 2.30 p.m. I open my paysheet and deposit $1000 into my bank account. On the 20th of December at 2.30 pm, I feel blessed to be part of a productive team that moves my area forward. I lead a productive team that is conscientious and has fun. I appreciate my money energy that represents my value to a conducive institution. I am engaged in excellence that has grown who I am. I am the best version of me."

"Well done, Turquoise, that's a great start, and we can work on your goal to be even more specific to include your every desire so that you see the possibilities for you to and seize relevant opportunities that will serve you. Setting your goals and securing them on your future timeline will help your brain focus on who you need to be to take the steps towards your goal. The more you look for opportunities to be part of a more conducive workplace, the more of them you will see, and you will be able to choose your choice for your change from the many possibilities available to you," says Connie.

Connie gives Turquoise space to think. Turquoise takes a deep breath, and a smile creeps onto her face. Then she nods for Connie to continue,

"If you stay the same, then I need to remind you about workplace rust that stems out from boredom, monotony in routine, or even just a sense of dissatisfaction. You may experience a drop in motivation and performance. That's right. Be careful because you may even develop mental health issues like depression and anxiety," Connie gives Turquoise space to process the information.

"I don't think that I want to go down the road where work issues lead to mental health issues," says Turquoise with a tear in her eye. Connie nods and continues,

"You told me that Beastie is continually making fun of you for drinking lots of coffee, and you said that you limit your coffee intake to two cups a day. And he criticizes you for overeating chocolate when you provide chocolate snacks for team meetings. Is it okay if I add that it seems that Beastie is effectively perpetuating your feelings of being found out and not being enough? You have experienced the process of suddenly losing responsibilities, which can lead to bore-out, which is a term that captures feelings of distress arising from the monotony of a job that neither challenges nor provides any sense of meaning. It can lead to severe mental health issues too. There is research that suggests that too little or too much of something can lead to boredom and bore out."

Turquoise listens and thinks about Connie's words. Then the voice in her head brings her back to speak her thinking out loud,

"I can feel my confidence drop when that fear of I don't feel good enough makes me fear that I'll be found out. I always feel overwhelmed when the fear of being found out arises within me. And then I don't know how to be good enough in the Men at work misbehaving club. They want me and my staff to be innovative in moving backwards, and I don't know how to do that, and then they clumsily do the micromanagement thing. That's when I feel confusion build within. Putting that aside, I wonder if I can change my focus to find other possibilities that will support me."

Connie listens and then says,

"What if you changed your problem from being innovative to move back in time to seeing it as a challenge of change moving towards their desired outcomes as directed?" asks Connie.

Turquoise stops to breathe, looks down at the floor, and then bends down to scratch her ankle. Turquoise lets out a loud sigh and breathes. She sits upright again. She looks up at the spot on the wall above her and in front of her. She basks in the calming feeling within the silence, and then she continues,

"I think that I can see their directives as a challenge instead of a problem, and that feels better because I can imagine that I own the challenge and I let them keep the problem," Turquoise sighs loudly and says,

"I label myself as an empath which means that I can be mindful of and understand how others feel about an event or situation. I also believe that empathy is about me being able to identify and understand my values and beliefs. I also think that having empathetic passion is all about identifying and understanding other peoples' values and beliefs and sensing things from their perspective through their view of their world.

Daniel Pink says that- "Empathy is about standing in someone else's shoes, feeling with his or her heart, seeing with his or her eyes. Not only is empathy hard to outsource and automate, but it makes the world a better place." https://www.brainyquote.com/quotes/daniel_h_pink_521933#

And I know that a red-necked quorum is an individual group working dysfunctionally in my world. I have discovered that my level of thinking has the flavour of love and connection a couple of steps above the rednecks' level of thought. I understand that the rednecked level of thinking is aggressive and insular, where the rednecks think that it's all about them. It's about getting what's theirs and staying on top. Forgive the pun, but the red necks in my institution are designing their world to be on top and sometimes on top of many, and I sense that they believe that it is nobody else's business. They are arrogant, and together the redneck quorum builds that muscle to prove it. They flex their aggressive intimidation muscle daily to control the environment around them and confirm their might. I can see it, and I know what it is like to be manipulated and feel obliged to be the fall guy, just like I internalised and owned the blame for not being good enough with Lincoln and Golly. They can manipulate each other to be incompetent, and to me, that means that their world is about to collide with my world with them efforting to make my world a worse place. I do not want to compromise my values and beliefs to be one a red-necked participant. I don't want to sell my soul as Beastie has sold his soul to be part of the redneck quorum."

"Well done, Turquoise, for coming so far," congratulates Connie and then Connie says,

"I have watched '*Who the bleep do you think you are*' and '*The secret*'. I understand from my viewing that Quantum physics says that we are the past, the future, and endless moments of now. All possibilities are available to everyone, which means that they are available to you and me too. What do you think?"

Turquoise says,

"That sounds generous and kind. I like that, and I think that I am ready to think about my contribution choice of information towards making another goal. I desire that I now choose my choice for my change. In three months from today, I can see that I will be working in an environment that best aligns with my values. I feel worthy and confident to connect and contribute to growing my team, who are moving forward because we are empowered to add value to make our work world better and better every day. I focus on the endless opportunities available to me and choose to know what they mean for my choice for my change. I sense my self-confidence build. I know I am worthy, and I now trust my actions to take me towards my preferred outcome because I know that I can keep choosing until I find opportunities and possibilities that work for me. I feel excited to see that I can learn from my experiences, knowing that there is no failure, just feedback. I can design a mind map that centres my desired outcome and links the goals that show the steps for me to keep me on track. I will know when I attain each result because I feel happy working in a supportive and exciting environment where I can easily taking care of my commitments."

Turquoise stops to think, then says,

"I believe that I have realised that I need to let go of the need to impress others. If I don't require their approval to be the best version of me, I can be my best version. If I sense the goodness in me, then I can find it in everyone. When I embrace who I am and share it, I believe that I attract an appreciation for who I am. I can write the best version of my resume to position me to apply for jobs where I fit."

Turquoise sits quietly for a moment and notices her excitement wane, and then she says,

"I will even try to see the divinity in Beastie, Grim and Slippery Jim, but sadly, the image of goodness within Beastie, Grim and Slippery Jim evades me."

Turquoise stops and rubs her forehead, squints her eyes and sits bolt upright, then leans forward and continues,

"I will keep trying to discover the divinity or goodness in Big Red, Beastie, Grim and Slippery Jim. I now know that I can change my focus to believe in myself and immerse myself in being the best version of myself to meet the challenges ahead.

I think that the following Be the Best Version of You, four-step process may help me.

Step one. Focus on process and not on perfection. If I change my focus on process rather than perfectionism, I will attract success because I will choose to move forward. I can focus on my feelings of worthiness to trust that I am doing the best I can to meet the challenges. If I focus on my worthiness, I can move forward. When I'm doing perfectionism, I am not moving because I get stuck in making the perfect solution for my problem, and there is no perfect solution. I believe that we are perfect in our imperfections, of who we are and all we do in life. If I focus on perfectionism, I may experience anxiety because I spend my time worrying about what is ahead of me and then I never arrive at my success point, and I don't want that outcome. I make that mean that I will choose to focus on what I want instead of thinking about what I don't want.

My second step will be to let go of the need to be right. Sometimes when I feel that someone has wronged me, I expect an apology. I still feel the need to hear an apology from Beastie, Grim and Slippery Jim. I know that I will be waiting for a long time. I know that I can feel better if I permit myself to release the need to be right and forgive them for their rightness. I would forgive for my sake, and they don't even have to know. I will try to forgive them for the dirty way my doctor said that they had treated me."

Turquoise stops to ponder. Turquoise chews her bottom lip and then says,

"Okay, I will acknowledge that everyone sees the world differently, and they may be too into themselves to know that they have wronged me? If I forgive them for their actions, I will stop my resentment from bleeding into my life now, and in the future, if I forgive myself for resenting them, I can clear my negative feelings. If I let go of my ego's need always to be right, I can restore my happiness and contentment. If I practice happiness and joy, I will take those feelings with me, and I can choose to leave behind the feelings that I let Grim and Beastie generate within me.

My third step would be to let go of the desire to gossip. Right now, I know that the quality of my life depends on the conversations that I have. I'll change my focus to talk about things, not people, to brighten my life to have an optimistic or more positive outlook on life. When I talk to myself, I can challenge myself to see everyone's divinity and step back to observe their behaviour. I can be the observer and watch for behavioural code. How cool would that be?

My fourth step would be to let go of the past. I know what has happened and understand how to change my feelings towards those events, but I can't change what has happened. I can change my beliefs and emotions associated with my past experiences and bring my new beliefs into my plans for my future. I can change my belief around my experiences. I cannot change what has happened. I am who I am right now because of my past experiences, and for that, I am grateful. I will do the best I can to enjoy now and be present. I will build my resilience muscles to survive my place right now and in the future.

Now that I have direction, I can focus on where I want to be, what I want it to feel like, and sense that I am already there. I can imagine where I am, what I am wearing, how I'm feeling, what I'm thinking about, what I hear myself say to others and myself. I can concentrate on being in the moment."

Turquoise pauses to breathe and sip her water,

"I now know that the law of attraction says that it will give me what I am. If I ask how I can give, then the universe will give it back by how I will receive.

How many times have I heard that you need to focus on what you want, not what you don't want, or you will get more of what you don't want?

If I focus on coming from my heart space, not my headspace, to be my authentic self and feel that happiness space, I can feel confident to back myself. It's like I will have my unconscious mind on board with my conscious mind, and when the unconscious mind and conscious mind align, I have a happy mind that works to give me the best to be the best. I can then listen to my logical thoughts and use my creativity at the same time when I can connect my heart space and headspace to decide to take on board those thoughts that will serve me. I believe that it is essential to connect my intellectual intelligence in my brain with my emotional intelligence in my heart when making decisions instead of following the manipulating orders from others. I refuse to do anything like tampering with ballot boxes just to please a potential sponsor."

Turquoise emotes and intellects, and then she takes a slurp of water. Turquoise takes time to sit back in her chair and relax until she is ready to speak again,

"How about I tell myself that Grim, Beastie and Slippery Jim are doing the best they can. I can choose to think positively, and then my positive thoughts will bring me positive outcomes. Like the American Indian child who was asking his grandfather,

"If we have a good bear and a bad bear inside us, which one will survive?" The grandfather answers, "Whichever one you feed."

I, too, can choose which bear to feed. If I nurture my awareness, even more, I can make informed choices that serve me, serve others, and serve the greater good.

I now know that I can't change Big Red, Grim, Beastie and Slippery Jim, nor can I influence and manipulate them as the rednecked quorum does for them. I can only change myself and decide which of my inner bears to feed because I can't feed their inner bears. Only they can."

Turquoise pauses once more. Time passes, and then Turquoise fidgets in her chair to make herself comfortable, takes a sip of her water and then continues,

"I know that when that little voice in my head sends doubts or takes my focus from being confident to self-doubt, telling me that I can't do this, or they may win because they are misbehaving or they are stronger. I know that it is my ego talking to me and doing its job of trying to keep me safe that is safe from change."

"Excellent work Turquoise," says Connie,

"I agree about our egos intentions. Let me share what I have learned. Our ego hasn't evolved and still thinks it's keeping us safe from the sabre tooth tiger. Those thoughts of doubt that come to you have an intention to keep you safe with the purpose of keeping you the same. For example, if I were to choose to stay indoors or go for a walk, my ego would guide me to staying indoors to keep me safe from the scary elements out there, like an extinct sabre tooth tiger attack. Yes, well-intended. My ego will also kick in if I walked alone in the bush and saw a dark snake across the track ahead. My ego would pump my adrenalin and set the fight, flight or freeze reaction in action. I know I would be running so fast that you wouldn't see me for dust. That's when I would be saying thank you ego for saving me from a snake bite. We have evolved into a different lifestyle where we no longer have to stay in our cave to escape the now extinct sabre tooth tiger attack. We can choose to change and confidently break out of our comfort zone because it seems to me that today our greatest fear out there is economic. Turquoise listens and nods. Turquoise sits quietly, deep in thought for a bit, then Turquoise says, "My greatest fear is the red-necked quorum, but I refuse to stay inside to hide from them. I just want to leave them. I intend to listen to my inner voice and respect that it intends to keep me safe. I will listen and then choose what serves me and thank my inner voice for speaking with the intent of keeping me safe. I will thank my inner voice and tell my inner voice that I will confidently follow my choice of direction to move forward. I believe that my self-talk is vital because I need to discern the difference between staying the same to keep me safe and finding the courage to decide what is best. Do I hang in there and conform to survive, or do I find the courage to leave and flourish?"

Turquoise rubs her hand on her thigh, wriggles in her chair to sit in a more comfortable position and then continues,

"I can draw on my past to understand the experiences that contribute to my story. I remember when I was a school student travelling to school on public transport. I remember listening to a woman yell at a man to let him know that his behaviour of exposing himself to her was unacceptable. I watched with awe as she beat him with her closed umbrella as they stepped onto the train station platform from the train carriage. He was bending over with his hands covering his head, and she was standing tall and upright, stretching towards the heavens as she brought her unopened umbrella down on his head. He became more bent and smaller; she became more elevated and exploded with extraordinary strength. At that moment, my belief in patriarchal dominance was turned upside down. I learnt then that there was strength in finding my inner matriarchal courage.

I may need to take an umbrella to work with me to listen, give credit where credit is due and just whack Beastie when he takes credit for other people's work and claims it as his success. Metaphorically speaking, of course. I know that I can be courageous and believe that I can win over them. I can trigger that belief by visualising a closed umbrella coming down heavily on them when I say a strong no because I don't want to be part of them."

Turquoise smiles and contemplates her idea. Turquoise continues speaking,

"Even though I love adventures, I prefer some certainty of knowing that I have another job before I leave here. I have a plan to stay until I can leave on my terms as I deserve. Then I will make an effort to imagine the divinity in Beastie, Grim and Slippery Jim. In the meantime, I will strengthen my resilience by imagining my umbrella strength and know if the lady on the train can beat evil with the swipe of an umbrella, so can I stand tall and choose to believe in myself and know when to say no and when to yes. When I imagine the umbrella, I too will know my strength."

"That's right, master your mindset to know that you do not need to take on board responsibility for others actions and their mindsets. Change your approach and listen but don't internalise their negative personal messages. Imagine that you open the clear perspex umbrella that will protect you from them. You can imagine that you watch their communication and sense their messages hit the perspex and ricochet right back at them. Don't forget to remember that you can forgive, and remember not to forget so that you are prepared if they do it again," says Connie.

Turquoise nods and smiles. As Turquoise walks towards the door, she turns to thank Connie for their session.

The chair in the coffee shop that Regie was sitting on was bowing under his weight. Turquoise smiles and greets Regie,

"It's so good to see you."

Regie rises from his chair and hugs Turquoise. They were long time work friends and now shared similar interests in artistic creativity and artistic expression. They sit opposite each other at the small coffee shop table. They order coffee. They spend time chatting and then sit quietly for a bit.

Regie looks at Turquoise and smiles when he says,

"We've been friends for six years now even though I left the industry two years ago. I can't tell you how free I feel. I just couldn't do what you are doing anymore."

Regie rises from his chair and asks the waitress directions to the bathroom. Turquoise watches him as he walks away.

"Regie is the butterfly that has emerged from the Chrysalis. He wants to share his transformational success. Life for him is excellent. No longer is he suffocated in the cocoon of rules, regulations, and processes of the institution that he had left. Like Turquoise, Regie liked the adventure of life and connecting with people through whatever means presented itself. He wants to see the same transformation for me. From the welfare worker to the yachty, chasing his Nirvana on the open seas was undoubtedly a shift," whispers Turquoise quietly to herself. She then sits quietly, not thinking of anything in particular.

Regie is Turquoise's long time friend and breaks into her silence when he says,

"Why don't you just reinvent yourself."

"Yeh, yeh that would be a good idea to reinvent me," answers Turquoise,

"I have to adapt to sameness every day. If only I had the foresight to flee when the going was good. It wasn't my fault that I got caught up in the insidious restructure that was a staff review that no one knew was happening. It seems to me that the natural attrition of staff isn't working fast enough. I have survived three amalgamations in my youth, but now that I am older, I guess it is my turn to take that golden handshake, and I am waiting for the gold." Turquoise smiles broadly, then she says,

"The persuasive freedom of basking in what the big wide world out there is offering is awe-inspiring. And then that feeling of fear envelops me like there was a little voice telling me that no job means no money coming in, and then what? But I need to be released from the chains of regulations and processes just like you, Regie."

Regie sits opposite his friend Turquoise who is lamenting that her job change is out of her control when she says,

"My values of integrity, loyalty and respect, are compromised because I have lost respect with men in charge misbehaving. I think that they are foolish and somewhat duplicitous." Turquoise stops to take a deep breath and think somewhat, and then she asks,

Do you mean reinvent me as the observer?" asks Turquoise. She pauses to think again, and then she says,

"As I think about the next time that image of Beastie and his cohorts enter my thoughts, I can imagine that I am the emotionless observer watching me watch them on the big screen in a picture theatre. I can watch them move across the movie screen and out the other side because I am now an emotion-free observer watching the movie and no longer an invested participant. I notice how much better I feel knowing that I am choosing to not immerse myself in the Beastie and his cohort's emotional story. Can I do this again?" Turquoise asks.

"What if the fearful feelings come up again? Will you be able to become the emotionless observer at will," asks Regie.

Turquoise stops to take a breath and starts talking again,

"Let me tell you how I stop feeling fear and scared?

I practice deep breathing. If I breathe in deeply through my nose and then breathe out through my nose, I will stimulate my vagus nerve. The vagus nerve interfaces with the parasympathetic control of the heart, lungs and digestive tract. I wonder if you know that it's the longest nerve of the autonomic nervous system in the human body. I practice deep breathing to stimulate the vagus nerve because its purpose is to facilitate feeling better. I follow on with rhythmic breathing because I find it helps calm me, just like the undulating movement of the sea waves calms me. I remember experiencing that calm feeling in my scuba diving years. The underwater currents would soothingly sweep me along, and the waves on top lifted me and carried with their swells. When I went with the flow, I experienced that calm feeling as I concentrated on the sea waters ebbs and flow. When I focus on my rhythmic breathing, I feel the same calmness. I become aware and listen to my intuition, and I believe in this instance, the messages from my senses tell me to run.

Run and run fast away from the stress and don't look back may come to mind in this scenario. I have learned that stress triggers cortisol hormones and adrenalin hormones. These hormones are released from the adrenal glands to take blood to my muscles, preparing me for fight or flight. I don't want to stay and fight because I know that long term stress can cause a decline in cognitive functions, and I would need clarity of thought to influence my feelings to focus on keeping myself safe from them. Grim and Beastie stress me. They are out to get me and celebrate my downfall."

Turquoise stops to take a sip of water and then continues,

"I have learned that long term stress can affect concentration. I am beginning to feel the effects of long term stress because I swear that my mind is rusting out with boredom. Grim and Beastie have taken away my responsibilities. I feel like I am moving backwards, which is boring because I miss the stimulation of the challenges moving forward. I will need to manage the rust in the short term until I am ready to leave for greener pastures.

I have learned that I can have boundaries. I can build my boundaries to permit myself not to take on others problems. I can have a place where I can say no to intruders like Grim and Beastie, and when I do, I know they will react because I know that saying no will stimulate their wrath even more. If I let them cross my boundaries, they will threaten my sanity and my safety. I will need to fight them even more because they are growing into super-strong bullies. I think that I can find the strength to honour my boundaries. If I practice deep breathing followed by rhythmic breathing, then I can trigger the sympathetic nervous system. When activated, it sends a flash of hormones to boost the body's alertness and increases heart rate, sending extra blood to the muscles preparing me to run. I can be calm to postpone my flight and delay my fight response until I am ready to leave on my terms and choose my choice for my change."

Regie smiles and recites his favourite Dr Seuss quote,

> **"Dr Seuss: You have brains in your head, you have feet in your shoes, you can steer yourself in any direction you choose, you're on your own, and you know what you know, and you are the one who'll decide where to go.** (https://www.goodreads.com/quotes/22842-you-have-brains-in-your-head-you-have-feet-in)."

"I love Dr Seuss, and this quote makes me think that positive thoughts create positive results. How many times have I heard that phrase?" Turquoise asks herself, and then she looks over at Regie and says,

"Thanks, Regie, for our clandestine meeting. It's great to see that you're happy now that you have freed yourself from the rigidity of the rules and regulations working environment. Good stuff."

"Your time will come. In the meantime, plan your run so that you can go with the flow and then look forward to that time when you are free. I've enjoyed meeting with you for a catch-up, and now I need to go," says Regie.

Regie and Turquoise say their goodbyes and promise to catch up again soon.

The next day Turquoise finds herself sitting with Connie. Turquoise says,

"I caught up with an old friend and my former work colleague, Regie. We had coffee and a chat. I felt lighter after sharing stuff with him. Regie's parting words with me were to look forward to the day that I would be free from the rules and regulations, and I guess he also meant free of my men at work misbehaving. And yes, I do have something to look forward to down the track. I learned that I can reach for something bigger and better to give me a reason to live and trust the world."

Turquoise stops to take a breath and then shares a smile with Connie. Turquoise continues,

"I remember learning from you that When you don't trust the world, then your world fills with inescapable stressful memories of helplessness and hopelessness that may become encoded in your immune system and bones. That is when you can create embedded beliefs through your early memories. Your memories can become embodied in your blood and immune system at a cellular level. You know, you can replace them with opposing memories by looking at yourself in a mirror and having a conversation with you to change the meaning of your memories. You can tell your reflection that you are in a safe and secure place, and you can tell yourself that the world is a safe place. Repeat these affirmations ten times each to tell your mind to look for the change. The more you look for change, the more you see change. If you have back pain because you feel unsupported, look for supportive people, and you will see people you can trust. Look for evidence that all is well in your world. Know that when you pick up your phone and it works each time, you can feel confident and grateful that you can trust your phone. If you organise to meet a friend for coffee and your friend is there to meet with you, acknowledge and appreciate your friend's reliability. Gratitude is a key to feeling better and better, don't you agree?"

Connie listens and then adds,

"On the flip side, be careful what you let into your world. If a movie or the news is ramping up the dangers in your world, then turn them off. Too much exposure to ramped up dangers can give you a false sense of risk and trigger emotions around trauma. You may be verging on experiencing Grim and Beastie trauma because it seems that you are the butt of their dirty doings."

Turquoise thinks for a bit and then says,

"I get what you're saying. I acknowledge that I am still learning, and I am learning how to change my focus to believe that I have a strong sense of self-value that progresses me to choose a healthy sense of belonging in my selected future workplace. I can work with my memories to change how I focused on helplessness and hopelessness to focus on feeling empowered and confident. I can change the meaning of those memories to make them mean that I feel supported and have a sense of belonging while being trusted to make decisions independently. I can support myself by looking for evidence that all is well in my world and bring that feeling of all is well to consciousness, to acknowledge and to appreciate."

Connie listens and watches as Turquoise becomes lost in her thoughts. Connie sees a mischievous smile creep into Turquoise's face and then hears Turquoise speak,

"I wonder if you read an article written by PRIVAATEI, citizens keeping an eye on the government # stalking the truth, which said,

"There is something in the water in North Queensland. A council executive manager was allegedly skinny dipping with a female co-worker during work hours. There certainly appears to be a trend developing in a far north Queensland Council and indeed local government. **www. PRIVAATEI.com.au**

m.dailymercury.com.au reported on 11 December 2018 that a skinny dipping manager has officially parted ways from a Far Northern council more than a week after he allegedly took his female co-worker skinny dipping. Another article in the Cairns Post warned people that a big saltie was seen lurking at the far north boat ramp."

Turquoise stops to take a deep breath and then says,

"My men at work misbehaving would feed the female co-worker to the big saltie crocodile. Hiding the evidence would ensure the preservation of their jobs, and they would do this in the spirit of conserving the wildlife. That's how screwed up my men at work misbehaving are."

Connie listens, and then Turquoise says,

"The former article triggers my thoughts of Men at work misbehaving. If I were the judge and jury, I would throw the men at work misbehaving off the boat ramp and see how they like to swim for their lives. However, as tough as they seem, I doubt that they would be digestible."

Connie listens then says,

"Okay, it's time to stop wingeing. I know that we all do it. Now is your time to stop. Wingeing comes from our mind or our ego and not from our truth. Our mind can draw on past experiences and react. If we become a slave to our mind reacting to our historical past, we will experience a stuckness in that past event. Stop whingeing and stop permitting your mind to react whilst it reflects on your past experiences. Leave your past behind and be loyal to your soul and live in the now. Life is happening now. Yes, you can learn from your past and plan for your future, but right now is where you experience life because life is happening now, and you can choose from the many opportunities that surround you to create a new you. You are limited only by your imagination. Use your imagination to make yourself a new where you see the many available opportunities. Choose your choice for your change and just let karma take care of them. Do not bring them with you."

Turquoise stops for a moment to catch her breath, and then she says,

"I can decide to leave and choose a different workplace where I will be able to serve. I want to be part of the team where I can contribute towards moving forward, and that may mean that I decide to change to a different industry altogether."

Connie smiles and congratulates Turquoise for changing her focus on what she wants instead of what other people want for her"

"What else have you learned?" asks Connie.

"I have learned to look for and know my desired outcome. Now that I can elicit and understand my values to align with my goals to change my focus to change the thinking that changes my emotions to feel self-confident even more, I know that I have the confidence to take action," says Turquoise.

"Excellent," says Connie, "I believe that you are ready to leave the old that has been forcing you backwards to a new where you can spread your wings to propel you forward to be the best version of you."

Turquoise nods and says,

"I believe that sitting with myself as my best friend. I am enabled to take 100% responsibility for all aspects of my life. I can back myself to design my course of action, trust myself to have the self-awareness to choose what is best for me and have the flexibility to change what doesn't work and work with what does work for me. And as I believe in myself even more, I can feel the sadness, anger, and fear of being found out fall away from me. I can feel the peace, love, and joy emanate even more strongly and colourfully from within me. When I am aware of my heart connecting with my headspace, I feel supported and sense that I can be the best robust version of me for the world to see. I can take on the challenges and restore my self-belief to know that I can be the best version of myself.

And as Turquoise learns to recognise her strengths by finding her intrinsic values around connecting with people and having variety in her job, she discovers that she can make profound decisions. And as she aligns her decision making with her values, she feels her confidence build and her capability grow. And as she realises her successes in working as part of a team with people to move her actions forward, she realises that moving away from toxic environments opens doors for her to embark on yet another worthy adventure.

Turquoise kicks back and says,

"I love being a scuba diving instructor and travelling parts of the world, exploring to explore all that underwater has to offer me. I assist others in appreciating what under the water has to offer whilst teaching them about the importance of loyalty that will keep themselves and their buddies' safe."

Turquoise stops to take a breath and then excitedly says,

"I'm very excited that I get to be part of a team that breeds loyalty to each other, and I get to lead a team and take responsibility for my safety and other people's safety at work in and out of the water.

I am required to continue learning to keep my qualifications current, to maintain my licence and excel as a leader and educator. I just love working in an environment where self-respect, respect for others and respect for my environment are mandatory for maintaining integrity, safety, and education to ensure that I move in and out of the water safely. I feel like I have found my tribe in my happy place where I belong. I can connect with people and connect people with the inhabitants of the underwater world. Every day I experience the great outdoors' adventure and wonder what adventure I will encounter each time I splash into the water."

CHAPTER SEVEN

Debbie – The force of destruction; from hurt to healing

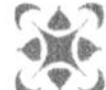

"And as I acknowledge Debbie as the Alpha female, I am inspired and respect her as a force to reckon with as she is powerful, leads with destruction, makes her mark, and is gone. She terrified me, she strengthened my resolve to match her strength, and she wore me out, leaving me feeling sick, sore, and very wet.

Intellectually I know that Debbie is just a cyclone. She is just a low-pressure system formed over a sea-surface temperature that rises to more than twenty-six degrees centigrade. Cyclone Debbie generated destructive winds with wind gusts that measured more than 300 kilometres per hour, bringing with it downpours of a metre of rain, thunderstorms and lightning," Echo tells her mentor, Alison. "Debbie scared me as much as bushfires terrify me, and even some workplaces can make one's blood run cold."

Echo flicks her hair off her face and then continues,

"I remember hearing a quote about how changing your perception can change the meaning you give, and I did that with Debbie. When she was a cyclone, she was a threat to my family and me and then she was given a name, and that is when I changed from running for cover to wait out the storm and check the devastation afterwards to standing tall to challenge her blow by blow. I hung onto those glass sliding doors as though I were fighting for my life.

"When you change the way you look at things, the things you look at change." – Wayne Dyer (https://www.goodreads.com/quotes/758151)"

Alison smiles and listens when Echo continues her speak,

"I remember feeling terrified as we drove into a T- intersection where bushfire smoke appeared from the left and then the right. Fifteen-year-old me froze until my driver turned right, then I curled into the foetal position in the back seat. I remember that I closed my eyes and held my breath because I was too scared to move because that was all that I could influence or control, or so I believed. I stayed like that until I felt confident to peek out of the backdoor's car window and see the blue sky above. When I sensed the smell of smoke dissipating, I allowed myself to feel confident that we were safe. I remembered that the fire for me was even more frightening than Debbie's destructive winds and a metre of rain falling on top of me all at once." said Echo,

"Now, when I look back in time, I see that I could have responded differently. If I permitted myself to respond instead of reacting, I would have decided to decline my mammalian brain's effort to keep me safe and freeze in fright. I would trust my thinking brain to lead me to feel the courage to have confidence in my driver to make the right decision to turn away from the fire.

So if I can change the way I look at the threat of a bushfire and a destructive cyclone to find my confidence and courage to work towards keeping me safe, then I can do that in other parts of my life too."

Alison listens and then asks,

"What else do you have to tell me?"

Echo thinks quietly then responds,

"Debbie was wet and windy, and she was challenging, even more, challenging because she had a name. Her breaths were strong, vicious and potentially disastrous. She threw her breaths in dangerous spurts past me. She threw her breaths of wrath like the narcissistic woman who was determined to get her way, and I had learned to take the challenge. I remember yelling aloud. Yes, I can do this. She will not get the better of me. And as she threw her wrath at me, I became even more determined to match her wrath. I told her again that she wasn't going to beat me. I was controlling what I could as I hung onto my front doors even more tightly, opening and closing to ease and influence the pressure."

Echo sighs deeply and takes her time to take three deep breaths and then continues,

"I remember thinking that a name made Debbie so much more real. I shifted from being the person I was to feel my muscles strain and adrenaline rush because I became determined to win in this situation. I'm not normally competitive, but this time I was up for the challenge of beating her. Normally I would go with the flow and experience the ride or hide, but this time I drew on my learnings from escaping the bushfire. Like the driver who decided to turn right, I could decide to be protective or do nothing and be exposed. Debbie blew so hard that she had stolen the roof from the bathroom that was my designated safe room, and I watched the tin fly down the street. I became even more determined to find the courage to hang on to my doors. The doors that provided a protective barrier between me and the wrath of her blows out there. If I decided to let her take my doors, I would be her victim and exposed to her blows with nowhere to hide." gasps Echo.

Echo sits upright in her chair as though she is proud of herself for overcoming her fear by looking inside herself and knowing how she can influence herself.

"I remember so clearly thinking that my courage grew exponentially." Echo smiles then says,

"I remember yelling out loud to Debbie and telling her in no uncertain terms that I was going to win and that she was not going to beat me. Debbie, you can blow me down, but I will get up and go another round. You watch me. You give me wrath, and then you will receive my wrath because what you sew you reap.

Water flowed in around the windows, through the holes in the roof that Debbie had stripped bare. Water flowed through gaps in the roof where Debbie had lifted the corrugated iron sheets and under the corrugated iron walls where they used to meet the floor. I held on tight and yelled from the room filling with water,

You're not going to win this round. And as I felt my arms ache and experienced Debbie blow harder, I sensed my self-doubt trying to make an appearance. Part of me was hanging on tight when another part of me tried to negotiate my safety. If I run into the bedroom, I can pull the mattress from the bed and drag it into the smaller bathroom. I can use the mattress as a protective covering to keep me safe. Debbie can take my roof and blow my house down, and I will be safe hiding under the mattress. I thought for a moment and realised that both parts were trying to keep me safe. I could see that my roof was lifting even more, and Debbie had taken my front security doors. If Debbie takes the glass sliding doors that I hold onto so tightly, she'll blow and push the ceiling upwards and away. I imagined the upstairs falling downstairs and then the walls falling in, and then I imagined that she would blow us away. Debbie's wrath motivated me to continue the challenge to influence what I could to keep me safe. I continued to open and shut the big glass sliding doors to regulate the pressure. I would then close the doors and hang on tight as Debbie blew even more strongly as she tried, even more, to take my doors from me."

Echo stops to ponder her courage and confidence that she found to meet her challenge. Echo smiles and then continues,

"I can't influence or control the wind and the rain, but I can influence how I choose to respond, and this time I chose courage, and then I found my strength. Corrugated iron tin sheets blew up and down the street, some from my roof and some tin sheets blew from other places. Debbie dropped a metre of rain that night. The rain fell through the holey parts where the corrugated iron roofing material was missing or lose. The water rose through the gaps where the walls met the floor, and water poured through the window frames' cracks. No matter how quickly we mopped, the water soon grew in-depth on every floor surface. I felt surrounded by devastation as I helplessly watched my terrified dogs who roamed the house looking for somewhere to hide from all the water. The feel of wetness rose against their legs. The sounds of the roaring winds terrified them as their bulging eyes looked around them. Their tails were between their legs, and with eyes wide open, they searched the ceiling, trying to dodge the water falling from the heavens. I watched on helplessly as my dogs' ears flattened against their heads, protecting them from the loud noises of wind and the roars from water falling from the sky," Echo sighs with tears in her eyes and then continues,

"Debbie showed her strength, and her voracity propelled me to finding mine. I found the strength to go with the process. I went with the flow of what I couldn't control and controlled what I could. I found my purpose. One of my dogs, who is the size of a small Shetland pony, decided to lie on his raised dog bed above the waterline. He lay with his legs crossed and his head raised. He was focusing on me with pleading eyes like he was relying on me to protect him. Debbie roared and blew like she wanted to blow my house down. And as I observed my dog, I yelled that Debbie was not going to win any round. In this battle, she was threatening my family and me. I found the incredible strength to work the heavy front glass doors to beat her," Echo tells Alison,

"Cyclone Debbie smashed the tree that had then regrown even more abundantly. When confronted with massive winds, the tree had demonstrated that it could go with the flow of the blow bending it one way and then the other. After time passed, so did Debbie and took her hard-nosed psychopathic violent, obsessive, manic behaviour with her.

The decimated tree engulfed in corrugated iron sheets drew on its strength to recover and rejuvenate to be even grander than before. It was like the tree had stood firm and shed its dead leaves to make way for an abundance of new growth,"

Echo stops to rub her forehead and move into a more comfortable position in her chair. Her eyes light up as she says,

"I can change how I see things, and I can do this by modelling the tree that rose from the ashes after being smashed by Cyclone Debbie. I can model the tree to believe that I can regrow even more strongly. I can build my strength to believe that it is possible to have the flexibility that will allow me to move with the flow of the storm in any part of my life. I, too, can find that strength, courage and determination inside me to be who I choose to be, to do what I need to do to have the strength to build my resilience muscle to be greater than before."

Echo thinks for a moment before continuing her soliloquy,

"If I control my thoughts, which create my feelings and how I choose to emote to the world, then I will be able to influence my life to feel empowered and own my courage that I can decide will remain within me.

And as I overcame my fear of Debbie, I found that my strength grew, and I knew that I would win. I am still here, and Debbie is only a memory."

Echo takes a deep breath and wriggles in her chair, and then begins talking with Alison once again.

"I chose to save the glass doors, which put me at risk. If a flying missile hit the doors, the projectile would strike at the same speed as the wind, which measured 300 kilometres per hour. It would possibly have sent shards of glass right through me. I chose to ignore that risk and overcome the fear to build my resilience even more. When the threat receded, I acknowledged my power that created my empowerment to build resilience and strength to win the battle. If there is a next time, I can remember the steps that I took to weather the storm and save my glass sliding doors, and I can draw on that courage, strength and resilience to do it again whenever I choose."

Echo stops to take a breath and smiles before continuing,

"I have experienced cyclones in the past but not at the ferociousness of Debbie."

Echo lets out a loud breath as though she is modelling Debbie's strong windy gusts and then continues,

"I won against Debbie, even though the journey was challenging. I learned to challenge Debbie even more so because she was a cyclone with a name."

Echo thought about the tree, then continues,

"If I choose to be like the tree that had lost its leaves to the big blow, I too could rebuild, restore and regrow. I now know that I can recreate my feelings because I recreated my sense of exhilaration when I survived the bushfire. I learnt that I can model others like the driver who decided to turn away from the burning bushfire to know that I can choose my feelings. I can feel empowerment, build strength, create new, choose my choice for my change, and be the architect of my life to shape me to be the best version of me. I can decide to stay to fight the storm or decide to leave. If I stay, I know that I can recreate my power within to recover, restore, regrow, or if I choose to go, I know that I can trust myself to choose my choice for change to keep me safe to live my dreams. My learnings are cross contextual in all parts of my world, and I can do the same in any environment that beckons me.

I grew my courage when I held on to the glass sliding doors despite Debbie's big blows. My arms hurt, and my fingers cramped, but I still held on tightly. The doors were the boundaries that divided my safe space inside my home with the life-threatening cyclone Debbie out there. I had a light behind me inside my house whilst black darkness enveloped the world outside. Debbie pushed and pushed as she blew her devastatingly 300 kilometres per hour winds at me. I focused on making myself hold and secure my sliding glass front doors. I decided to strategically open and shut the glass front doors to manage the pressure build and drops because I knew she would pass even though she overstayed her visit to tease and scare me. Just like the emotions that darken within me, if I stay with them without a story, then they too will pass." "Yes, eventually you're going to recover from those emotions that have been troubling you because all things pass eventually," says Alison.

CHAPTER EIGHT

Dulce – working for the Corporate Psychopath; from hurt to healing.

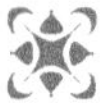

The Crocodile is biting, the Crabs are following, and the mangroves are beckoning

Dulce's hands are sweating, and she senses her heart pumping faster.

"I have coped with drama, trauma and life-threatening illness, and yet I fear Cyan, the narcissistic, psychopathic Crocodile that some call the corporate psychopath." Dulce stops talking to take a deep breath before continuing,

"She wants to meet with me again. I don't want to wonder what she has in store for me because whatever I do is wrong. Whatever word I write is wrong. Whatever I think is wrong." Dulce pauses to catch her breath.

"Why is it that some people who swiftly scale the corporate ladder feel the need to disempower the level of support staff below them to the point of creating a dysfunctional workspace?" Dulce asks Edith, her coach and mentor.

Edith sits quietly and observes Dulce fidgeting in her chair. Then Dulce takes a deep breath and continues,

"You know Cyan, who I call the psychopathic narcissist, and others call the corporate psychopath, seems to have lost sight of the big picture and the outcomes she once aspired to. I often sense that Cyan is confused because she seems to have lost her clarity around where she's going and how she will get there. Cyan complicates her progress by deliberately setting me tasks and then whenever I am close to finishing the job. She tells me that I'm doing it incorrectly. Because I am using the wrong words. And she tells me to rewrite and use the right words, and when I do, she tells me to do it again over and over. I have made a belief that she's obsessive about setting me up for failure. Cyan often says that her obsessive-compulsive disorder motivates her perfectionism. I know that she's systems motivated and appears to lack emotional intelligence.

I know this because Cyan will identify the wallabies who are a perceived threat to her. I notice that the targeted wallabies are naturally strong thinkers who can see the big picture and know how to get there. Then she instructs me to fabricate situations where they are set up and targeted to blame for corrupt behaviour. It's like she is thinking with her reptilian crocodile brain mixed with a little mammalian brain where she thinks only of her survival. Then I am remiss because I just can't do what she asks. After all, the Wallabies deserve to feel valued for their significant contribution to the team. They should be encouraged to grow." Dulce sighs loudly and laments,

"Cyan is a challenge. That is all I can say," Dulce sighs again and continues,

"It seems that when Cyan fears her perceived threats, she raises her stress levels, and that is when she defaults her brain function back to her primitive need for survival. Cyan waits, observes and knows when to snap up her prey like a crocodile and then spits out the leftovers and repeats the same behaviour for survival. I guess her fear is even more overwhelming than I first thought because she's past scaring people with her bark. I reckon that she has withdrawn way back from her mammalian brain, where her fight, flight and freeze response resides. She's gone down deeper into the primitive survival crocodile brain that is even more fearsome than pretending to frighten people with her bark and more threatening than her threat to bite like a dog. I think that I understand her stress levels soaring out of control because I have felt that too. I reverted to survival mode when I was overwhelmed with a life-threatening health diagnosis. I remember blaming events and people for stressing me, and then I decided to take responsibility to make life-saving choices for me. I took steps to survive, and so far, I have succeeded.

I feel a significant rise in my stress levels when I have to deal with Cyan. I feel like I lose all sense of ability when helplessness and hopelessness build overwhelmingly within me. I wonder if stress levels have drawn Cyan and me together, you know like you attract who you are. Even though Cyan's stress is drawing her down into the dark side, I like to think that I can see the lightness way over there in my chosen path leading me on my journey of life."

Dulce takes a sip of water and thinks, then says,

"In my opinion, Cyan pushes her stress levels even more because I believe that she is inspired to be the type of perfectionist who sets impossibly high standards for others. She sets her perfectionist bar so high even she cannot reach it, and that feeds her lack of confidence even more, which seems to push her further back into the darkness of her dark side. I see Cyan as narcissistic and antisocial, and when she chooses, she even has a dark, aggressive sense of humour. She seems to laugh with the corners of her mouth pointing downwards. I feel that she cares little about social norms and does not readily fit into the bigger social picture. I remember watching Cyan at a professional function drape her arm around any man of repute for support. And as I watched her drink from her upended bottles of wine, I saw her throw up before falling over, leaving me to clean up the mess and assist her out of the function room. When she's not drinking and draping herself over men because she is sober, she chooses invisibility. I know this because I have noticed that she will sit soberly and quietly in a corner out of sight, and still the corner of her lips droop downwards."

Dulce sighs loudly and takes a deep breath. She sits silently, for some time, contemplating her rant.

Edith jots down notes whilst she observes Dulce in her silence. After the silence, Dulce sits bolt upright, staring ahead at a spot on the wall just above her eye level. As she focuses on the spot, she sees more clearly and has clarity of thought when she says,

"Cyan seems to repeat that same behaviour over and over. Every time Cyan will overcompensate with too much alcohol consumption. It appears that she uses alcohol to hide her fear of being caught out because I think that she is naturally unsociable.

I know that Cyan relies on networking as a significant work component for her. Even in those circumstances, I sense that she chooses invisibility to hide her lack of confidence when there is no alcohol. It seems that maybe fear of rejection is overwhelming for her. Cyan is trying to fit in with the levels of command above her. Cyan tries so hard that she seems to pivot in the muddy place where the mud sucks her deeper into the detail. Each movement seems to suck Cyan down even more. Every time Cyan shoots me down, she tries to suck me down with her," says Dulce.

Dulce falls silent again as she sorts through her thoughts. She is no longer focusing on her own perceived weaknesses but Cyan's narcissistic, psychopathic behaviour.

Dulce lifts her eyes to refocus on that inspirational spot on the wall, and then she lowers her eyes and speaks,

"I remember that time I rang Cyan to let her know that I wasn't well enough to return to work, only to be told, do not return to work until you are resilient, and I meekly replied with an okay."

Dulce fell silent again, and then she felt anger rise within her. Her stomach churned, her breathing became a little tricky, and she wasn't sure she could speak, and then she did,

"Resilient for what? She didn't even ask if I was okay."

Dulce sits quietly for a few moments longer and then says,

"You know Cyan is like a Crocodile focusing on its prey, waiting with jaws wide open ready to snap, with its army of Crabs waiting by her side, to feed them the leftovers. It makes me feel claustrophobic and closed in like a prisoner held against my will. I need to get out of this mangrove that is the institution that drives the Crocodile to hold me captive so she can chomp me up, spit me out, and destroy my life entirely as I know it now." Dulce takes a couple of deep breaths and then says,

"Think I need to escape the mangrove before it becomes my burial ground. I have always got my jobs on my merit. No one hands them to me on a plate. I apply, I participate in the interview and participate in any other required processes to prove my worth before confirming my suitability for the jobs that I do."

Dulce sighs loudly and then continues,

"I want to say that I respect Cyan, but I am just scared of her. My focus was on the fear of Cyan, and it didn't enter my mind to fear the institution's culture that encouraged behaviour like Cyan's behaviour. I remember feeling shaky that time when Cyan asked me a question. That's right, a question, oh no. I went into meltdown. I felt my heart pounding in my chest, my hands instantly felt clammy, and my forehead was a horrible sweat. At another time in a different place, I was asked what the team had planned for a festive event. I usually responded with vitality and excitement because I love to share possibilities and conversation, but when Cyan asks me a question, I hesitate to answer because I am damned if I do and damned if I don't," Dulce stops to take a breath and then continues,

"I remember a time when I thought that Cyan was fact-finding to set up her workflow for her yearly budget planning. I remember thinking that maybe this time, the correct answer would be that she is looking for yes, we can do it without a budget. I sensed that Cyan doesn't care about my answer because she consistently focuses on shifting monies to support her spending rampages with public funds. Cyan spends just within the accepted boundaries or not as she believes that she is bulletproof."

"Did you have a project in mind?" asks Edith.

Dulce smiles, a mischievous smile,

"For my project, my team and I would like to tame the Crocodile. I need to say up front that we have an active imagination. And as we see that our first action would be to create an alibi, our imagination would lead us to make a to-do list, and we would include items of importance. For example, we need to find somewhere to hide the bodies. The first step would be to call a team meeting to establish rapport, communicate clearly to know that we are working towards the same outcome. The second step would be to identify the steps to take and work out our contingency plan. The next step would be to ensure the congruency of the project for consistency and to know that we are on the same page. The key is to have team rapport and the behavioural flexibility to work together towards the desired outcome. It is essential to know that it is ecological and good for you, others, society, and the world and then go forth confidently. The first agenda item for the plan would be to discuss the shopping list, including shovels, tarps, and lime bags. Shovels to dig a big hole. Lime to dissolve anything. A tarp to hide the dig."

Dulce sighs and takes a sip of water, and notices Edith staring with her mouth open, so Dulce says,

"Okay, we'll build her a comfortable underground room with padded walls so she can't hurt us any more and can't hurt herself. Our contingency plan would be that if our original idea doesn't work, we could arrange a professional development event further south to throw her unkindness into the vats of acid, dissolve her negative behaviour, or venture north and take her to the other mangroves. And as that resident crocodile chomps her up and spits her out, as she does with us, we can sit back and sink deeper into celebrating the success of our plan. The best thing would be that we approve of our proposals."

Dulce stops to draw breath and then continues,

"I guess my plan represents how I feel. I get sick of hearing that Cyan says that your staff are so emotional that it didn't happen like you said it did. I wouldn't have done that to you. It is your fault. I never did that. You are the one who is lying, and you should have told me because that is illegal, and the list goes on. I just don't get it. Why do I have to feel guilty," sobs Dulce,

"She deserves to feel what we have all felt."

"Stop." says Edith," And as you sit there, you might have noticed that burnout comes from overwhelming stress and can lead to mental health issues like depression or anxiety. You may have already noticed a drop in your performance and lack of motivation. Burnout is a result of a process, not a single event, and Dulce, you mentioned that Cyan consistently targets you, and each time you feel more and more distressed, is that right?" asks Edith,

Dulce nods, and Edith continues,

"As you sink deeper into process, you might notice that process becoming a habit. Maybe that habit will leave you feeling depressed or experiencing anxiety set in you like ice sets."

Dulce's face pales as she quickly interrupts,

"I don't want that to happen to me. I don't want to be fearful for my future, and even more, I don't want that fear to become part of me. Help me, please, Edith."

Edith agrees to help and asks,

"What is there to learn from feeling guilt when Cyan constantly targets you?

Dulce bites her bottom lip and blinks rapidly. Then Dulce answers,

"When I feel guilty about my performance, I think that Cyan senses my vulnerability to target me even more,"

"What else have you learned?" asks Edith

"Dulce says, "I have learned that I look to Cyan for approval."

"That's right," says Edith, "How do you know that you are doing a great job?"

"I know when I feel empowered, confident and happy.," responds Dulce.

"And where do you find those feelings?" asks Edith.

"I find those feelings of empowerment, confidence and happiness inside me, and that is when. I feel like I am the most important person to me in my world. I feel exhilarated and awesome," responds Dulce.

"If you learn to trust your thoughts that create your internal feelings and emotions, then you wouldn't have to associate into those old fearful emotions that you find out there. You wouldn't have to use energy to make up revengeful stories to make you feel better. How will you feel when you can release yourself from those emotions that used to arise when you referred to Cyan's opinion of you?" asks Edith.

"I will be elated, and I will feel lighter," says Dulce and then she takes time to immerse into the new thoughts that make her feel different. Dulce is sitting quietly as her curiosity stirs. Edith continues,

"Change your Mindset. You can, you know. Did you know that your conscious mind is responsible for only 5% of your daily thoughts, feelings, and behaviour? And as you sit there, you might have noticed that your conscious mind requires a great deal of effort and uses willpower, critical thinking, systematic analysis, logic and reason? You might have noticed that you can use the conscious mind to access the unconscious mind. We form our habits in our unconscious mind, and that's where our emotions and memory come from, where we can find creativity, imagination and make instant decisions. Our unconscious mind is responsible for 95% of our daily thoughts, feelings and behaviour. You can choose your choice for change in that 95%, and you can do this even more rapidly using self-hypnosis. I am a trained hypnotherapist, and I can guide you in your use of self –hypnosis. You just have to ask."

Edith gives Dulce some thinking space to process, and then Edith continues,

"Imagine holding 2 million matchsticks in one hand and taking 126 matchsticks from the pile and see how many you have left to choose another completely different 126 matchsticks. Imagine how many times you could choose a different 126 matchsticks. If the matchsticks represent information and each matchstick represents different information, imagine how many times you could choose different information on which to focus. Each time you choose different information to focus on, it can change your thoughts to change your feelings to mean something different and lead you somewhere else. You can choose your choice for your change by shifting your focus from one lot of information to another. You can make changes in your strategies, focus, values, beliefs, purpose, and environment to change your view of your life effectively. I won't tell you that learning is easy and powerful, and it's happening now. When you have 2 million bits of information hitting your senses at any time, and you only take in 126 bits because that is all that you can absorb, then there is a lot left to choose from to change your 126 bits of information," says Edith.

Dulce responds,

"I think I get it. If I shift my focus to focus on different bits of information, then what I focus on can change the meaning that I give that different information. I can then choose to feel confident about my choice of response. If I change my focus from people-pleasing based on external feedback, I can choose to seek the power within me to back myself to let Cyan keep her critical words. If I focus on changing what Cyan's words mean to me, I can choose to know that Cyan's words are self-criticism because I now know that her words are a projection of how she perceives herself in her world. When she spits her words at me, I understand that I can now choose to stop to take a breath and then decide what to think to create the feelings I choose to support my decision making and influence my choice of response. I can choose to rise above the victim cycle and be the observer. And as I permit myself to disassociate as the observer, I discover the power that I have always had within me. Then I see myself as the confident and integrious person that I choose to be. I can believe in me to formulate a framework around my decision-making that will give me the certainty I need to make decisions moving forward. When I believe in myself, I will discover the power that lives within me to effectively back myself and protect my feelings from Cyan's ubiquitous attacks. When I shift my focus, I can change the meaning of my thoughts to choose my feelings that affect how I emote to the world out there, and I can change how I see my world and even change my emotions to change my life. and that is how I can change my mindset."

Edith nods and then listens as Dulce says,

"I can focus on what I can control within me, and I choose to go with the flow or not with what happens out there. I can choose what to think that will choose my feelings. I can choose to be an observer and stay out of other people's drama. I can change my mindset from thinking that I will be found out or being judged. I can choose to know that I can engage in non-judgemental feedback to improve each day. I can know that I am good enough to back myself when I become the observer and dissociate and make Cyan's criticism of me be about her, and then I don't need to take it personally. If perception is a projection, then her criticism and judgement of me is her criticism and judgement of herself. It's about her and not about me," exclaims Dulce excitedly and then says,

"When I choose to take Cyan's criticism as feedback, then I know that I don't fit with Cyan as part of her team. I feel that I just don't fit into this institution because it has its strong processes, even down to every word you write when I think about it. This perfect culture is not necessarily good for my brain because it has a culture of always being right. This culture expects its employees to obey rules right down to each word used to communicate. I know that I can make informed decisions to take responsibility for what I feed my brain, and I choose creativity and logic instead of always being right. This institution is a very seriously compliant and challenging environment for me. It is a powerhouse of problem-solving and outcome-driven, where a conscientious psychopath like Cyan and her cohorts can easily hide. It seems to me that this is a place that is attracting even more narcissistic corporate psychopaths.

I know that I have the patience to listen and nurture, and I sense that I'm gifted with strong emotional and social intelligence. I can get along with anyone, and I find it easy to create rapport. I don't get along with Cyan no matter how hard I try. I'm guided by how I feel, and working here with Cyan does not feel good. Does that sound right to you because it makes perfect sense to me. I just don't fit into this institution.?" Dulce takes a breath and then pauses to ponder,

"This place has so many hiding places, and I'm transparent. I remember a good friend telling me that people don't get the opportunity to gossip about me because I tell them all. After all, I have nothing to hide and that makes me vulnerable here. Should I be hiding my understanding and empathy in the many hiding holes that surround me?"

Edith gives Dulce space before reciting a quote that Edith remembers and recites,

"One doesn't have to operate with great malice to do great harm. The absence of empathy & understanding are sufficient. Charles W. Blow (https://www.goodreads.com/quotes/628593)

It seems that Cyan can manipulate people because she knows how to use guilt and flattery to get what she wants, and if she lacks empathy and understanding, then she won't feel a thing, so to speak."

"Oh my goodness, that sounds like Cyan, and I don't want to be like her," exclaims Dulce.

Edith nods and continues speaking,

"Do not let her draw you into her drama. Make space between you and Cyan to keep yourself safe for the time you have left working with her. Because you can't avoid her, make sure that you keep your emotions in check and present a calm demeanour at all times. Remember to stop and take deep breaths, to interrupt the energy flow between you. Stop her from manipulating your emotions to control you. Don't show that you are intimidated. Know that Cyan will attempt to scare you to dominate you. From now on, stand your ground in an assertive manner and record and report incidents.

Whatever you do, please do not buy into her stories because she will tell you her victim stories and quickly turn them around to persecute you as the victim. Everything will be your fault. Turn the conversation back on her by pointing out her flaws to disarm her. When she tries to blame someone else, turn it around to her and ask,

"Are you doing okay?"

Or

"I noticed that the meeting stressed you. Are you okay?"

Opt for online communication whenever you can because if you have it in writing, you can report it with written back up. Cyan can't charm her way into a better deal because writing to communicate with emails will weaken her efforts to communicate face-to-face. Ignore Cyan's criticism of your writing and write it down. Change your fear of her to her fear of you.

Above all, you must maintain a healthy mental attitude and maintain self-care to survive the time before you move to another institution. Come and see me or ring me when you need to. Be strong."

Dulce wonders about being strong because she has frequent dreams telling her to get out of the mangroves before the Crocodile chomps her up and spits her out to be crunched even further by the Crocodile's minions. The Crabs, who are the minions, are always waiting to devour the rest of Dulce.

In her dream, she can hear Edith's voice,

"If you stay, you will lose prestige. You will lose credibility, and above all, your self -confidence will plummet. Your body will warn you to get out by creating ridiculous health issues. Your mind will spin into overwhelm. You will have the feeling of loss of purpose. Even worse, you may begin to question your very existence. Only you know how far someone can push you."

And then Dulce wakes in fright.

"I have dreamt this dream so many times it feels like it is part of my reality," says Dulce. And Dulce burst into tears.

"I try so hard to do what Cyan wants, but I don't know how to please her. I feel helpless and hopeless at the same time. My shoulders hurt, my head hurts, and everything hurts, "sobs Dulce.

Edith waits whilst Dulcie catches her breath. Then Edith listens whilst Dulce compares herself to Albert Einstein's fish. Dulce says,

"Everybody is a genius. But if you judge a fish by its ability to climb a tree, it will live its whole life believing that it is stupid." Albert Einstein.
(https://quoteinvestigator.com/2013/04/06/fish-climb/)

I don't want to be the fish that is required to climb the tree every day. I feel that Cyan expects me to be like the fish and sets goals at the top of the tree. And that is where I feel helpless and hopeless.," sobs Dulce.

"Dulce, you have told me what you don't want. Can you tell me what you do want?" asks Edith.

"I want to feel worthy and appreciated. I want to be confident and optimistic to leave with a confident and optimistic outlook to know that I will work in a job out there waiting for me. A job for me where I fit and belong. I want to live in my genius," says Dulce.

"What I am hearing is that you want to change your feelings from helplessness and hopelessness to being optimistic about attracting the same in a new job. Is that right?" Asks Edith.

Dulce nods and then listens to Edith say,

"May I share with you that you have a conscious mind that is like the tip of the iceberg and an unconscious mind that forms the larger part of the iceberg that is hidden under the seawaters. Your unconscious mind is responsible for preserving the body, it stores memories, and your unconscious mind organises memories and represses negative emotions. Your unconscious mind presents memories to your conscious mind to release negative emotions. Dulce, you can change your feelings from helplessness and hopelessness to optimism by breaking through your fears that you mentioned earlier of not being enough, not being loved and being rejected at an unconscious level. You can do that most effectively using self-hypnosis. How does that sound?"

Dulce pauses to think some more. She remembers a time when she placed her attention on her thoughts that attracted her sad emotions. Dulce remembers feeling sad and amazed all at once when she watched The Lion King three times. Dulce felt sad three times, and three times tears rolled down her cheeks. She knew it wasn't real because it was a movie with special effects. Each time her energy in motion drew on the familiarity of her emotions when watching sad movies, she cried each time.

Dulce mutters,

"If I can generate the sadness feeling three times from familiarity, I can choose to change my initial emotional response to respond differently to outside stimuli. I know that not every feeling I have is correct. I know that I can challenge my negative feelings and emotions unless I am standing in the middle of the road with a semi-trailer speeding towards me. I will then need to acknowledge the danger and take flight towards safety. That means that I can choose to let my feelings control me or learn to control my feelings. My feelings and emotions are not facts, and if I change, they can change how I see things."

Dulce looks at Edith and says,

"I have given Cyan the benefit of the doubt before only to find that she is still callous and preys on me and uses her cunning to play with me. She exposes me with unsettling images on her computer and waits for my response. That's when I feel that she is trying to upset me so she can watch my reaction. I have to say, though, that I feel proud of myself because when I recently looked at Cyan's computer screen as she asked, she showed me an offending post online and told me to look at it. I looked, but I didn't comment or give away any indication that I was unsettled. I had decided that it was her problem, not mine, and at that moment, I chose not to own it. She didn't like it. Cyan pulled her thin lips taught. Her face reddened from the bottom of her neck up to the top of her cheeks. I turned away and couldn't help smiling. One win to me. I now know that I can change the confusion in my head by changing my thoughts that I use to create my feelings and emotions that will change my life."

Dulce thought for a moment, wrinkling her forehead and pursing lips, and then she says,

"I can try to understand Cyan's motivation to understand her behaviour. Her badgering is relentless, and I now know that I don't have the energy to live life on her terms. I need to find the courage, even more, to look after myself. I need to trade Cyan in for a better model, but I know she is not going anywhere, and if she does, then there will be another corporate psychopath somewhere in the structure that will follow her and hide as she has. Maybe not in her position but someone higher up in the ranks.

If I stay, I know that I can't influence her, but I can control my thoughts and feelings to understand that I can change myself. I understand that I can choose my feelings and emotions to handle her and make the best decision for me moving forward. I understand that I can do this by changing my focus from how her behaviour affects me to how I will respond to her behaviour. I value integrity and will apply my value to me and be my own hero."

Dulce sits with a wrinkled brow and chews her pen for a while. She then removes the end of the pen from her mouth and takes a deep breath, and says,

"If I could choose, I would like my supervisor to be reliable, friendly and know that I have my supervisor's support in times of change or crises. I am adaptable and can adjust my behavioural profile to serve others, but I can't change her behaviour. However, I can design a version of my ideal supervisor and change from familiar to unfamiliar. I can be that person to attract that person.

I have discovered that I adjust my behaviour to meet my environment's demands whilst working for the narcissistic, psychopathic Crocodile. I now know that I felt confused because I didn't know what I needed to take towards the institutions end goal. I acknowledge that I haven't set boundaries that serve me. I wanted to experiment with not setting limits to see if that would strengthen my conformity. I efforted to survive in her rules and regulations environment. The more I try to conform, the more I grow my feelings of insecurity and confusion. I spent my time trying to please her, and it was me who needed to find the courage to value me."

Edith stops Dulce and says,

"If you focus on only pleasing others around you, you will feel extremely exposed and vulnerable and open to attack."

Dulce stops to think again Then continues,

"I am resigned to give myself the space to discover who I am and to know what I need to change to honour my authentic self. I will find my courage to be the architect of my life moving forward. I have discovered the intrinsic values to me and those values that help me design my ideal life moving forward. My courage leads me to sit with my Mentor to process forgiveness. Clearing my attached resentment towards Cyan frees me to remember my experience working for Cyan without feeling the feelings that hurt me. My experience has already taught me to take back my power by changing my focus to change who I need to be to have the thoughts and emotions that will guide my decision to become the best version of me."

Edith sits with Dulce and supports her journey when Edith says,

"Think about how you feel. If you sense that you are gossiping or thinking negatively or contributing to drama, then acknowledge and say to yourself cancel, delete, clear. Then change your focus to choose your feelings of joy, fun and talking about things, change your posture to look the world in the eye,"

Dulce listens and wrinkles her brow, and Edith says,

"Well, try this. Slouch forward on a chair, let your chin drop to your chest and feel what you feel. Now sit up straight, look the world in the eye, and feel how different and confident you feel. Imagine sitting forward looking directly at the person to whom you are listening to let them know that you are interested in them and connecting with them."

Edith observes and asks,

"How did that make you feel?"

"I could feel a big difference in the stances," replies Dulce.

"That is a beginning. Step out of your deep hole into your shine by stepping into your power. Find the courage to change what doesn't serve you and find what does serve you to serve others and serve the greater good," advises Edith,

"How many of us have gone through drama and sometimes trauma and come out the other side. You can control what you can control within you, to respond instead of reacting.

Listen, then take a deep breath and then decide to respond or not. Your thoughts create your feelings and emotions that are your life's energy. You can change your past emotions that build on each other through Timeline Therapy to change your emotions at their core. You can change how you feel about your memories and change your feelings to change your life now."

Dulce interrupts and says,

"I can use the forgiveness process to free myself from past emotions. Essentially, I can experience giving up the thoughts around what the past could have been, so I don't drag those emotions into the now and my future. I can then free myself to move on with my life. If I can find the root of my negative decisions and limiting emotions from my past experiences, I will discover a place where I can change my focus to change the meaning of my past events through forgiveness. I will then be empowered to choose my change even more quickly and succinctly using self-hypnosis techniques. I will feel my power to change my focus to change my perceptions of myself and my life. I can then choose to believe in myself and back myself to find another work environment in the same industry. A place where I can fit and be my authentic self, a place where I can contribute and feel valued and a place where I can connect with people to have a team impact."

Dulce set about applying for other jobs.

"I know that you are wondering, and it's a good thing to wonder because there was no one to keep you safe out there in the mangroves. And as the Crocodile waits and watches for your predictable behaviour, waiting for the right time to attack, you feel uncomfortable, and you know you are out of your depth. You can not change the Crocodile's behaviour, you can not change the mangroves capability to be what it is not, but you can change you. And as you change your focus, you can change your thoughts that change your feelings that change your behaviour. Dulce, you can forgive the Crocodile for its transgressions to feel better about yourself, but you cannot change what the mangroves hide."

Dulce thinks for a moment and then says,

"I can acknowledge my emotions related to feeling attacked, forgive my attacker, appreciate the release of my negative emotions from my body at a cellular level and be grateful for discovering my peace. When I feel peaceful, I can find the divinity that is within all of us. And as I see the divinity in others, I know that forgiveness has worked. I know when forgiveness works for me because I always feel different when I have processed in the past. I remember feeling my courage to back myself and trust myself to do my best whilst seeing others' divinity. Believing in myself to stand up for me replaced the pressure of the previous feeling of my need to conform to my external environment."

Dulce stops to think. She wrinkles her forehead and shakes her head when she continues,

"I have discovered that my values are misaligned with Cyan's values and with the institution's values that are stiff with conformity and unforgiving. I believe that Cyan's values are around being rigidly right and confusing to cover her fear of incompetence because she does not know how to apply what she knows. So if I choose my future choice for employment to align with my values, I could find a work environment where I could create empowerment to create even more success.

So if I stay, I sense that I would discover the mangroves' wrath because I don't fit into their values,"

Dulce stops to breathe deeply to ground herself and then continues,

"And as I can push myself to comply and be rigid to write the correct words on paper, I would force my energies into overdrive. I would become tired, I would feel my muscles stiffen, and I could even become ill. And as my body warns me of the stress created by my workplace's mismatching, I could get sicker until I stop to listen. And as I hear that my values mismatch my institution, my body would warn me even more. I don't want to get to that point."

Dulce stops to take three deep breaths to quiet herself. She sits quietly and begins to speak,

"If I can rebuild my confidence levels, I can once more choose a fair fit workplace. I can decide to elicit my values and confidently support myself to move onto a place where I fit. A workplace that aligns with my values where I can build my strength to create growth. To do that, I would use my courage to back myself and trust myself to do the best for me whilst focusing on others' goodness. Believing in myself to stand up for me feels like the freedom that I have been seeking. I feel like I can replace the pressure of the previous feeling of my need to conform to being beaten up for the transgressions that were happening out there in my external environment where I had no control or influence."

Dulce stops to take a breath and continues,

"If I change my focus to change my perception by controlling my thoughts, that change my feelings inside me, I can change my narrative to choose my feelings to influence how I emote to the world out there. I can change my life's story to feel confident that I can go with the river's flow pushing away from the mangroves towards the vast ocean full of choice. I can experience that ocean filled with opportunities and possibilities to choose my change choice. When I focus on my area that I can influence, I can confidently experience the water flow and its waves that promise adventure. If I choose what I can't influence or control and throw bad into the ocean, the ocean's rips will carry the bad away. I know the bad will ride the waves and come back at me two-fold. When I let that happen, I give my power away, and then the Crocodiles will have me in their vile clutches and drag me down the slippery slope into the depths of their world's depravity of blaming, shaming, and beating me up until I decide to run far away. So if I wait to run, I will then be scarred and limping forward in my life. And then I may become easy prey for the next Crocodile to feast on me. Those narcissistic, psychopathic Crocodiles like to build themselves up at the expense of others. Do I really want people like that in my life?"

Dulce wriggles in her seat to make herself more comfortable. She takes three deep breaths and relaxes into her chair. Edith observes Dulce focus on a spot on the high point of the wall. As Dulce sits comfortably, she closes her eyes and then continues,

"I can choose to let go of people, things in my environment and emotions that I no longer need in my life. I can choose instead to connect with like-minded people. If I am in the right frame of mind, I can seek out work environments where I can fit."

Dulce whoops a big, "Yes, I can," then she continues,

"I feel my feelings of excitement and happiness right now, and I choose just to sit and experience my emotions even more. When I close my eyes, I imagine that I am floating way up there and looking down. I imagine floating on the clouds above while observing everything happening way down below that no longer affects how I feel because I am too far away. I'm so far away that my work institution is just a pinprick in the scene below. I watch what I see below and see so much activity in so many various industries. So many options to choose my choice for change."

Dulce's eyes dart from side to side under her closed eyelids. A smile creeps across her face. She is breathing normally and mutters,

"I feel like I am watching a movie, and when I look down at everything that is happening down there, I no longer feel affected emotionally. There are so many happening people everywhere who are doing all sorts of stuff. It's so busy I am beginning to sense that overwhelm is wanting to creep into my consciousness. Declutter, Declutter, and Declutter some more."

Dulce sips her water and says,

"And as I decide to leave my current work environment's emotional clutter, I find that my confidence builds. My courage appears that supports me to find my courage to be a role model and have the confidence to create a business to help others achieve harmony by decluttering their environment as I did. I now trust myself to write my own marketing plan and copy that attracts enough clients for a successful business model because I know there is power in my writing."

CHAPTER NINE

Giselle –Working for the dragon narcissist; from hurt to healing

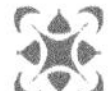

"I know that you are wondering, and it's a good thing to wonder because that means that you are learning many things, and all the things, all the things that you can learn, provide you with new insights and new understandings. And you can you know, can you not choose your choice for your change and know it's more or less the right thing to choose? You are sitting here listening to me tell you about changing your focus to choose your thoughts to change your feelings to know that you can. And that means that your unconscious mind is also here and can hear what I say. And since that is the case, you are probably learning, and it's more or less the right thing, that you can choose from the many opportunities available to you to design the life of your choice so you can be the architect of your life. You already know more at an unconscious level than you think you do, and it's not right for me to tell you learn this or learn that. That's right, you learn in any way you want and in any order. So as you breathe quietly and effortlessly at the perfect rate, you can let go of all tension. How would it feel if you discover new ways of thinking about the problem? And you notice, I mean, you really notice that you're starting to change now. Because sooner or later, you'll fix things, and sooner or later, you'll discover ways you've already changed. The more you search for that old pain, the further away it floats, and the more you learn to feel good again, the more enjoyable your life will become."

As Alicia continues her guidance, she works towards bringing Giselle back into the room. Alice gives Giselle the space to open her eyes, look around the room, move her body and then settle herself in her chair.

Alicia smiles and gives Giselle space to enjoy her relaxed feeling.

"So tell me, Giselle, how do you feel?" asks Alicia.

Giselle smiles and says,

"Wow, that was so good. I feel relaxed, and I am enjoying just sitting here. It's like a heavy blanket of discomfort has lifted and flown away. I can see more clearly now, and I feel a little more clear-headed."

"Now that you have found some clarity of mind can I ask what have you learned?" asks Alicia.

Giselle smiles and says,

"Listening to your stories has taught me so much, and I would love to share with you some of my relevant learnings. I now know that all possibilities are available to everyone and therefore they are available to me too. I know that there are resourceful and unresourceful ways of being, doing and feeling. I now know that I can influence what happens within me and that I can't control what happens outside of me, so I need to go with the flow or evaluate and decide what action to take. I need to apply my learnings to help with my decision making."

Alicia listens and then asks,

"I have an exercise to share with you that may further your clarity of thought around your decision making in your current work environment. Would that be helpful?

Giselle nods and says,

"Yes, please."

Alicia smiles and says,

"Okay. I suggest that you spend day one focusing exclusively on writing a list of things that have failed you and caused you pain in your current workplace. You can also list the mistreatments you have endured in your workplace and any other negatives that may come to you.

Day two, I suggest that you focus solely on writing a positive list of events where you feel gratitude and appreciation for others showing up to support you. You may include those times when you had job satisfaction, felt happiness, and the times that felt like you fitted in and felt like you belonged. Maybe there are some earlier events with Delilah to reflect on or some recent events that have escaped your notice.

Then dedicate day three for comparing, evaluating and weighing up the two lists for clarity around deciding to stay or leave. When you finish the process, you can write yourself a letter of reconciliation and purpose to create happiness in your future choice of a workplace to design a better future for you. You can imagine how your intention will promise how things will change for you in the future. You may choose how you would like to feel, how you would like to see yourself at work, and the conversations you would like to have. Imagine the change and feel the appreciation you feel and laughter you experience and hear, and describe your sense of motivation and aspiration."

Giselle listens and then asks,

"I think that I can do that. So if I do the three-day activity, do I then ceremoniously destroy the lists and the letter?"

Alicia smiles and nods,

"Yes, that's right."

Giselle and Alicia bask in the quiet, and then Alicia asks,

"Giselle, what else have you learned?"

Giselle says

"I have learned that I can change how I feel about the experiences that I focus on in my life that will change the meaning of the experiences to change how I respond to those life experiences. I think that maybe I will discover that the way I react to Delilah driving me mad is how I drive Delilah mad and then reacts as I would react.

I have learned that seemingly negative past experiences can create limiting beliefs that embed deep down. Maybe my limiting beliefs have influenced me to make negative decisions that affect what I think and how I behave in my everyday life. If I can change my focus to change my beliefs to influence my choice for change with future decision-making. Then I can choose to change how I feel about my past decisions and change the linked emotions to feel differently about those old emotions today. I can decide to leave my past feelings in the past. I know that I have the power to change my focus and choose the meaning I choose to place on that change that changes my thoughts that will change my feelings to change how I feel and respond to the world out there. And I can follow the focus changing steps as follows.

The first step for me to change my focus for a more positive future is to take **100% responsibility** for everything in my life. And know that I can change my perception regarding past events. Know that my power is in leaving the past in the past. Know that my strength is in living in the present moment and planning for the future."

Alicia smiles and says,

"Well done. What else have you learned?"

Giselle says,

"Taking 100% responsibility for everything in my life means that I can control my thoughts to change my emotions, which change my experiences. I have learned that integrity is my most important value from which I can design a loyalty boundary. And as I have a loyalty boundary for what I accept from myself, I can decide what I will accept and what I won't and then create a loyalty boundary for what I'm willing to receive from people out there.

As I change my perception of past events, I can leave my relationships that no longer serve me. I can change my perception of toxic work environment experiences into learning opportunities. And as I know that I can forgive other people's behaviour, I know that I will not forget so that I am more prepared to deal with their unacceptable behaviour now and in the future. I can build my boundaries for new experiences and current relationships based on my past learnings.

The Crocodile observes, plans and attacks his prey. I can model the Crocodile to take my time to observe their behaviour and to evaluate their value in my life. And as I use my more mature brain, I will know which relationships fit with me, which ones don't and which relationships and situations are redundant. I can choose to release redundant connections and keep those that are important to me. And I know that I can continue to test my decisions to act responsibly to serve me, serve others and everyone else.

So if I feel that significant people in my life compromise my highest value of integrity and break my trust, then I know that I can choose to make them redundant to my life and remove them metaphorically to make way for new relationships. I have a strong sense that I can declutter the old to make room for new. I can declutter workplace relationships to make way for something new. I can choose my choice of a workplace that changes my work environment to make space for new adventures and opportunities to connect with like-minded people as I grow in my life experiences."

Giselle sits quietly and imagines changing her thoughts to change her feelings that give her the emotions that lead her to experience the release of heavy feelings as she forgives herself and others and then continues,

"And as I forgive those who have transgressed me and forgive myself for my transgressions, I feel a shift within me. And as I realise that I can't change my past, I know that forgiveness means letting go of what I can't change in my past. Choosing to let go of past experiences means that I leave them in the past just like I have left my belief in Santa Claus behind me. When I forgive, I do it to let go of emotions that don't serve me now or in my future life. It doesn't mean that I forget the event. It means that I can choose my thoughts that create my feelings when reflecting on the event, and I can choose to do so without feeling that original heavy emotion. When I forgive Delilah, I know that I have forgiven her because I feel a shift in how I think about her. My fearful feelings for her have changed to feelings of indifference. I know now that I can confidently be in Delilah's presence for the duration as the unattached observer. I will see myself as good enough. And I now know that I can choose to move towards working in another environment where I can fit in and reignite my confidence to excel.

Now, I feel empowered to decide that I have the strength and courage to look for the divinity in everyone. I have a sense of growing my goodness inside me, and I understand that I will then see the goodness in others."

Giselle's eyes open wide, and she smiles when she says,

"Now I know that I can listen to the words of others whilst telling myself that they are their words, not my words. And I can choose to let Delilah keep her words. I can design my words as part of the architecture of my world.

The second step for me is to choose from the many opportunities available to everyone and therefore available to me.

And I now know that I can select from the many opportunities that connect me with people in a resourceful way. I can choose a work environment where I connect as part of a team to move forward. I feel empowered to choose from the possibilities that provide me with my choice of adventure and variety moving forward into another work environment whilst sustaining my emotional well being in my time left working for Delilah. I can learn to build my resilience muscle while working with Delilah and take my learnings with me to support me in my search for my workplace match."

Giselle feels happy that she believes that she is good enough to change her focus that alters the meaning of events around her to enable her decision making. Giselle feels her confidence grow even more and senses that she can believe in herself and says,

"I can design my steps towards my desired outcome through setting clear and specific goals that I can measure, that would make me accountable, that I can realistically achieve in my chosen timeframe. I can ask for career advice to match me with suggested career paths. Look at the choices that I have to choose from in my first search for suggestions that would fit my profile. These include Counsellor, Social worker, Local Government Councillor, Nurse, Middle

Management, Customer Service and HR Consultant. I can choose my choice for my change. I have so many career choices to choose from if I decide to change my career, and I can choose to focus on the learnings in my current situation whilst building my confidence and resilience if I choose to stay. I can choose my choice for my change.

The third step towards change for me is to discover operational values where my inner courage sits: to be aware and curious about choices, to know what works, what doesn't work, and to see what needs changing. Alice works with Giselle to elicit her top five operational values.

Alicia asks,

"What do you value?"

Giselle thinks and then says,

"Now that I feel calmer, I have a clearer sense of clarity, and I can say that even though the certainty of direction is important in my workflows, I do like variety. Knowing that I'm safe and keeping my team safe is even more important to me. I like to be acknowledged for my achievements, and acknowledging my team for doing well is important. Even more important for me is being part of a team and leading others as I would lead me. So I guess my intrinsic values are connection and safety. If I were an archetype, I think it would be the mother archetype with a bit of influencer of happiness archetype mixed with a perfectionist archetype, and that's where I will find my power.

I realise that integrity is important to me. I make my meaning for integrity include my truth, honesty, and respect. I also believe in courage because courage gives me confidence which gives me a sense of empowerment. I value good health both physically and mentally because being in the best of health will give me the strength to embrace life's opportunities. Good health energises the brain, and I believe that education is essential, too, because learning enriches my life. I permit myself to explore the adventures of life, knowing that there is no failure, just feedback. When I learn, I move and experience even more and grow abundance in every area of my life. Integrity helps me make decisions and design my boundaries, and courage supports me to experience life and be the best version of me. When I have good health, I can energetically follow my dreams. Education enables me to learn new, experience new, connect with like-minded people and grow myself more abundantly. I can grow my abundance through building self-esteem to experience my life's purpose even more. My values are from most important integrity, courage, health, education and abundance."

Giselle stops to breathe deeply, then she quietly thinks about her values choices.

"I now know my values are important to me and what they mean to me. They are the guiding light that I use to design my internal frame of reference to inspire me to no longer rely on external references to influence who I am. I can now choose my attitude of choice to create the boundaries that will keep me safe,"

Giselle says with excitement in her voice. She takes a sip of water and continues,

"And I know that connection and safety are my intrinsic values to show me where I fit. I know that my intrinsic and operational values guide and motivate me to find my authentic self, connect with my inner self, and explore how I care for others.

If I fit, then I can care for others instead of caring what others like Delilah think of me."

Giselle stops to take a few deep breaths. She wants to yell that she sees the light but thinks better of it, and then she continues,

"Hmmm. Maybe I just don't fit into this organisation as a whole. Just because it is proficient and works at exceptionally high levels doesn't mean it matches me. My natural or intrinsic values include connection and don't match working for people who are all about them regardless of others. My current place of work filled with rules, regulations and perfectionism seems to be a place where the narcissist or corporate psychopath could hide easily.

Maybe I just don't fit this institution that has a sole focus on rules, regulations and is authoritarian-driven to exclude people's well being. The same old, same old, limit my need for variety, and that's when I feel bored and unhappy. If that is the case, I need to leave, but I now know that I can choose another environment that would suit me better.

If I choose to stay, I believe that I will need to change my perspective to be open, flexible to bend with the rules, adapt to expectations, and let go of what I can. If I don't, I will experience a lot of resistance, like swimming against the river of life's flow. If I'm not flexible with my emotions and flow with the river of life, I will stop and stiffen. My body will become rigid like a dead twig that breaks from the tree when the wind blows. I believe that I can choose to stand still and let my external environment experiences happen. I can choose to let go of my resistance and flex with the flow of my external experiences. I can choose my thoughts that create my emotions that I can control and ultimately affect how I respond and react to the experiences in front of me. If I decide to become inflexible and slowly kill my career, then my dreams and health will be affected, which means that I would compromise my values.

The rules of the institution won't change. I believe that how I perceive those rules will help me adapt and recognise what I can let go of and what I can sense is of utmost importance to keep. If I am open to thinking differently, I will see things from a different perspective, and I will know what I can influence and what influences me. I will develop the art of letting go of emotions that don't serve me, other people's words that are not mine. I know that I can create feelings that support me.

When I let go of rigidity to be right, I can focus on what I can influence and what I can control, and then I can let go of what I can't influence. That's where I will find the clarity of thought that I need to develop the art of flexibility and the art of letting go. The person with the most flexibility will experience more, move more, and control their environmental influences."

Alicia's Mentor honours the silence that falls then adds,

"Can I share another of my favourite Lao Tzu quotes with you?"

Giselle nods and listens. Alicia says,

> **"A man is born gentle and weak; at his death, he is hard and stiff. All things, including the grass and trees, are soft and pliable in life, dry and brittle in death. Stiffness is thus a companion of death; flexibility a companion of life. An army that cannot yield will be defeated. A tree that cannot bend will crack in the wind. The hard and stiff will be broken; the soft and supple will prevail."— Lao-Tzu (https://www.goodreads.com/quotes.)**

Giselle wrinkles her brow whilst thinking for a moment. She then takes a breath and says,

"I do have the safety of tenure here, but I don't feel safe emotionally. If I could master my emotional reactions and choose how I respond to my thoughts, then I may find that emotion where I feel safe, and then I could survive for a while,"

Giselle stops and looks over at Alice for acknowledgement. Alicia smiles, and that is enough encouragement for Giselle to continue,

"I have learned that having awareness can set you ahead of your colleagues, and sometimes awareness can be uncomfortable and may be painful. I have learned to heal my painful emotions through a forgiveness process of releasing them from my mind and body. I know when I have changed an emotion through forgiveness. I can feel that something has changed because I can feel a change inside that something has changed. I know that I can reflect on a stressful situation without connecting to the stressful emotion. I can do this whilst I am preparing for my chosen change.

It is a weigh up to know what is best for me, best for those around me and best for my environment moving forward," says Giselle excitedly.

Alicia smiles and listens, then Giselle continues,

"And if my choice for change doesn't work the first time, I can make different choices until I have what is best for me, best for those around me and best for the greater good.

The fourth step is **understanding** that I can choose my choice for my change and have the behavioural flexibility to change as many times as I need until I achieve my desired outcome.

And I can grow my confidence even more, to change my focus to choose my choice of meaning that I choose for events happening around me that will influence my behaviour. Like the tree that bent forward, bent backwards and was stripped of its foliage during a cyclone, the tree spent time after the cyclone in recovery and then regrew even more abundantly, and I can plan to do that too. I can change my perception of my experiences and take my learnings from my valued experiences. And as I can forgive, I don't need to forget when I take my learnings in my plan to serve me now and in the future. If my plan works, I will continue doing what works, and if it doesn't, I know that I now have the resilience to get up and do something different. I know that I, like the Crocodile, can choose to spend time quietly observing, and I can observe functionally to observe my emotions and sit with my emotions until they pass because all emotions pass through me. Then I can choose my thoughts to focus on what will make my emotions. Life is a journey, and when I believe in me, I know that I can choose my choice for my change."

Giselle fidgets in her seat and rubs her hands on her thighs, and then continues,

"The fifth step is to focus on self-talk where I can build certainty in my self-belief to master my mind. When I master my mind, amazing things happen. I can tell myself that I have learned that I can be the architect of my life's experience and design the life of my dreams right now. And as I move towards making my dreams come true, I can trust myself and believe in myself to choose my choice for my change, and I can do this by choosing my thoughts to determine the feelings that serve me in life right now and moving forward. So if I harness my brain's power to connect with my heart space, I can be the excellence in my life and have the body language to reflect. I have learned that I can focus on self-talk to be different to make the difference."

Giselle stops to think and rubs her hand across her forehead when she says,

"I believe in myself and know that I can be different and be the architect of my life. I can navigate the fierce winds of life, even if they strip me bare and encase me with flying bits of corrugated iron that has been wrenched from neighbouring rooftops. Just like the tree that survived the wild cyclonic winds, I can find the strength within me to stand tall and steadfast against the roaring winds and flying sheets of steel. I remember that somewhere in my distant past, in one split second, a car accident stole my dreams and plans for my life as I knew it. I mourned, and then I rode the waves of recovery, reinvention and renewal. I lost part of me and then regrew anew even more abundantly than before, and I can do it again now. I can take my learnings from my past experiences and implement them into my life today. I now know that I have the courage to; recover, reinvent and renew. I can find the confidence to choose to discard what doesn't serve me. I can design my regrowth to be the person I choose to be, have the life I aspire to, and choose my environment to excel. I guess that is what is meant by taking your learnings from your past into now."

Giselle takes a deep breath then sighs loudly. She looks towards Alicia and says,

"If I could imagine that I dispose of those who hurt me and throw them into their mangroves for their Crocodiles to chomp them up and spit them out, I know that I would. That revengeful thinking drains my energy, and I want to energise, so I guess I need to find the goodness within them.

I could shift my focus to shine on other aspiring things. I could shine my focus to join a friend to work on activities that will distract and serve me. I could learn to build my fitness and participate in activities that will improve my health."

Giselle pauses, takes a sip of her water and then sighs loudly before continuing,

"And as I find my happiness within, I now know that's where I will discover unconditional self-love for me to be enough. I know that I can change my focus to choose my choice for my change. When I chose to elicit the root cause of my limiting beliefs and my negative decisions, I know that I can change the meaning that I give them, which changes how I feel about those memories. I learned to change my emotions around my negative thoughts and my negative decisions. And as I change my feelings towards my memories, I release and change the old and unhelpful patterns in my life. So if I can change my negative emotions, then I can change my negative behaviour patterns to find my courage to know that I am good enough to design new patterns as I journey towards the life of my dreams. That's right. I can now back myself to be the hero in my life and listen to the self-talk that encourages me to stand tall and choose my choice for my change. I can do this by making changes in small steps that will create a positive ripple effect to make changes easily towards being the best version of myself."

Giselle takes her time to breathe deeply and then continues,

"I have learned that I can change my focus to know that I can only control my inner self and my own emotions where I can find that peace that comes when you discover who you are and love yourself. I can choose to see the self-love in me where I believe in myself to influence my own life, and I have decided not to give my power away by listening to others who want to control me. So suck it up, Delilah."

"Well done." And then Alicia says,

"If you cannot influence what happens in the mangroves, leave the mangroves leaving the Crocodiles and the Crabs behind you and take your learnings with you. You can only influence how you feel, perceive what you see, hear what you hear and say what you think. You can influence your feelings, but you cannot influence how others think or create the emotion and feelings that make their behaviour. They can't control you. Only you can control yourself. Seek greener pastures where you look inside yourself to trust what you can influence in your life. Remember not to forget to remember Wayne Dyer's wisdom.

No one can create negativity or stress within you. Only you can by virtue of how you process your world- Wayne Dyer
(https://www.goodreads.com/author/quotes/2960)

You can choose to change your focus at any time. You have the power to give your thoughts meaning to influence how you feel, and as you do this, you can make the emotions that you show to the world out there. And as you can grow your resilience and assertiveness, you will discover that you can choose to survive in your work environment or find the courage to choose another workplace that makes you an even happier employee where you realise you can grow and build your strengths."

Giselle ponders her thoughts and says,

"So if I become even more curious to focus on my authentic self's peace, love, and joy, I will feel my strength grow as I sense that I can choose peace, love and joy as my building blocks to rebuild my self-confidence and belief in me. I can choose confidence to let go of my fears and choose to be empowered and confident in the dragon narcissist's presence by imagining the divinity within her and leaving her to think her thoughts and keep her own words. How will I do that?"

Giselle stops to think and then says,

"So if I change my focus to become the observer of the circlers in their toxic environments, then I can sit and watch them blame and shame as much as they like. If I waver, I can imagine that I sit behind an imagined plexiglass screen that deflects their blame and shame right back at them. And as I observe, I grow my self-awareness and my power to believe in myself. Then I can trust myself to change my focus, see their toxic environment as their design, and identify my environment as my design. I can resign my post as a people pleaser."

Giselle takes some deep breaths and tells Alicia,

"I have learned how to feel my emotions and become even more aware of my emotions when I sit with them until they pass as they always do, so if the dragon narcissist finds the crack to cut me deep and hurt me, I know that those emotions will pass. They will only linger if I make a story around them. And as I observe my emotions that linger through a story, I can choose to release them through a forgiveness process. And sometimes, I would need to forgive myself. And as I focus on my emotions, I can sometimes become aware of where in my body they present and learn what I need to learn from that part of me. I now know that when my back and neck hurt, I remember feeling unsupported and rejected. It was like the pain dragged my serotonin from me, and I would feel depressed or anxious. I believe that learning to manage my emotions will help me learn to manage my symptomatic physical hurts."

Giselle stops and scratches her head and then says,

"I have decided to believe that I can survive my time working here until I find something better if I become more self-aware of my feelings and emotions that I can control. Sometimes my emotions just pop up from somewhere within when I least expect them to, and I can learn to manage them also. I choose to believe that if I stop to breathe and concentrate on my breaths, I can respond as I prefer to respond rather than reacting to the triggers that my dragon narcissist sets. Creating space between receiving the information will give me time to think to manage my feelings and give me a choice to choose my response. And as I become aware of my feelings and emotions, I know that I can change my thoughts to change my focus to change my feelings and emotions to build self–confidence and self-esteem even more to more easily roll with the flow of the waves of life.

If I change my focus, I can change my story to a narrative that will make my future self proud. I now know that I can only influence my thoughts that create my feelings and how I emote to the world out there, which influences my actions. I learned that if I say I am and I have, I can influence what I can control, and I will attract what I can influence."

Giselle thinks about Debbie's wrath and how she hung around to play and taunt, and then she moved on. Giselle rubs her forehead, then rubs the bottom of her earlobe and then says,

"It seems to me that Debbie spewed her wrath for Echo to receive. Echo chose to fuel her strength using Debbie's wrath to stop Debbie's steal. While holding the doors and between the big blows, Echo stopped her thoughts and changed her story. Echo focused on feeling her wrath, her angry emotion, and observing its presence until it slipped away as all emotions do. So if I focus on those angry emotions without the story, then I know they too will pass."

Giselle stops to think some more and then continues,

"I think Echo respected Debbie's strength that fuelled her determination to recover, then regrow and rejuvenate just like the tree that Debbie's cyclonic breaths stripped and devastated."

Giselle stops to think some more and then continues,

"I now know that the freedom I have imagined is already within me. I have discovered that freedom in every part of my life is about feeling love for me. I believe that feeling loved is what we are all searching for, which means self – love, love for others, and being loved. We all need significance in our lives to feel that we matter, and that is why I need to feel that my contribution matters. If I flip the getting of significance to the giving of significance, then I can attract even more of that into my life and then I will make an opportunity to connect with like-minded people to know that I belong and feel loved."

Giselle stops to take some deep breaths and then continues,

"I think that I can create my boundaries to align with my values, and then I will know how to choose my battles because I will know what I will give myself permission to accept what I want and know what I don't want."

Giselle rubs her forehead and then says,

"I know that what is right for me may not be right for others. Every time I think about Delilah and this institution, I know that my concerns are that I don't fit, and I know that I need something to change for me to fit. I don't know if I make the change in my self-belief now or in a minute that will decide my next right step for me to take towards attracting the work scenario where I fit."

Alicia gives Delilah the respect of space to think and then asks,

"What if you did know the right step to take? What would that be?" asks Alicia.

"This something that I understand now. I need to understand my next step now as everyone can. The best thing is to know. Knowing my values and understanding my beliefs will provide a sense of what serves me and inspires me to build my understanding of worthiness and self-love even more. And as I find myself in a toxic work environment, I can maintain a positive attitude to plan and move towards a right fit work environment where I will come to belong, which will expand my sense of freedom. It will be where I will contribute my expertise and surround myself with like-minded people to give value through connection and contribution. The dragon narcissist can keep her cruel and heartless behaviour, and I can choose to take a breath and not accept her wrath, or I can choose to let her wrath fuel my energy to choose my choice for my change.

Knowing when to walk away is wisdom. Being able to is courage. Walking away with your head held high is dignity. (Southern Pinning) (https://www.lifehack.org/articles/communication/knowing-when-walk-away-wisdom.html)

Giselle chose to leave her job to take an opportunity of employment where she belonged with her tribe. A place where she could contribute and grow.

Giselle did leave on her terms, taking her learnings with her. Along the way, she sought the opportunity to re-educate herself and change her career choice. Giselle followed her heart to be self-employed as a hypnotherapist like Alicia to serve people seeking change in toxic work environments who want to choose their choice for their shift. She now connects with like-minded people whom she calls her tribe.

Giselle coaches her clients to grow as she grew, and then she grows some more to grow her clients even more. Integrity is Giselle's highest value that serves her well because now she feels loved, trusted, and innately knows that she is enough and even more. Giselle confidently gives her clients space to share their choice for their change and connects them with their unique hypnotherapy need. Giselle is satiated with variety in her job because every client is individual, and every client's need is unique. Giselle has learned to move her passions into a business.

"I have to flee the mangroves before the crocodile chomps me up and spits me out for her Crabs to eat my leftovers. They are doing my head in. I hate this toxic work environment where they do horrible things to me. How do I escape?" asks Giselle's third client for the day. Giselle sits quietly to observe and listen, then she says,

"People don't know all sorts of things, and a person may not know that you have all the resources you need within you. How quickly will you find these unconscious resources, and how quickly will you install them to feel much better. When you hit an obstacle, that obstacle can expand your change, and if you choose, you can make a change in all things in your life. And I wonder if you begin to change immediately. You can, can't you change your focus to change the meaning that you give to you in life to know that you can back yourself and you can, can't you? And as you think of how you'll apply this change of focus to begin your own internal search for meaning and as you trigger all the feelings, you remember where you were when you were deciding to take that job in the mangroves, with the crocodile and her Crabs. Where were you just before that? Now, as you think about your present situation in life, notice how many options you have now. As soon as you've had enough of this problem, you'll let go of it forever. Because sooner or later, you'll fix things and learn to back yourself and see you influence you and sooner or later, you'll discover ways you've already changed your perspective about the mangroves. Will you create some new behaviours before you leave the mangroves completely? Will you let go of the past before you heal all that sadness? Sooner or later, you'll fix things, and sooner or later, you'll discover ways you've already changed. How would it feel if you discover new ways of thinking about the problem? Every time you think of that old problem, then you'll feel a sense of humour and relief that it is gone. The more you search for that old pain, the further away it floats, and the more you learn to feel good again, the more enjoyable your life will become."

THE END

ACKNOWLEDGEMENTS

I acknowledge my mentors and trainers who have inspired me on my transformational journey.

I thank my family and friends for their support.

I am grateful for my friend Kate Wanchap who supported and encouraged me through my writing experience.